The All New Diverticulitis Diet Cookbook

A 3-way Nutrition Guide with 2000 Days of Safe and Delicious Recipes for Long-Term Gut Health | Includes 30-Day Symptom-Specific Meal Plans

Andrew Shallow

© Copyright 2024 - All rights reserved.

The contents of this book may not be reproduced or transmitted without written permission from the author or publisher. Under no circumstances can the publisher or author be held liable or liable for any damages, compensation, or loss of money arising from this book's information, whether directly or indirectly.

About the author

Andrew Shallow was born in North California in 1993. He is a chef and nutritionist from the USA. He graduated from the College of Nutrition and Food Science at the University of Carolina. This book is part of his passion of writing.

Table of Contents

Introduction 9
Chapter 1 10
Fundamentals Of Diverticulitis 10
What is Diverticulitis? 10
What causes diverticulitis? 15
Diverticulitis diet 16
Chapter 2 17
Introduction To Diverticulitis 17
The Clear Liquid Stage 17
The full liquid stages 18
The low-fiber stage 19
The maintenance stage 20
Chapter 3 22
Maintenance stage 22

1.	Delicious Oatmeal with Turmeric Powder	22
2.	Banana and Almond Butter Oatmeal	23
3.	Home Brewed Red Wine	23
4.	Ginger Carrot Soup with Turmeric Powder	25
5.	Ginger Soya-milk Soup	26
6.	Anti-Inflammatory Stir-fry	26
7.	Salad with Kale, Onions, and Apple Cider Vinegar	27
8.	Cucumber and Smoked-Salmon Lettuce Wraps	28
9.	Flax-Almond Porridge	28
10.	Blueberry-Millet Breakfast Bake	29
11.	Applesauce Burger with Spinach Salad	29
12.	Blackened Chicken Avocado Power Bowl	30
13.	Brown Rice Bowl with Turkey	31
14.	Spiced Mango Soup with Tofu	32
15.	Garlic Butter Chicken Meatballs with Cauliflower Rice	34
16.	Lentil Garbanzo Soup with Turmeric	35
17.	SPLIT Pea Soup with Spices and Coconut Ingredients::	36
18.	Tofu with Onion Sauce	37
19.	PULAO Rice Prawns Ingredients::	38
20.	POTATO and Rosemary Risotto	39
21.	SPICY Red Lentil Cauliflower Potato Casserole	40
22.	Lentil Pastries	41
23.	BUTTERNUT Coconut Red Lentil Soup	42

| 24. | CAULIFLOWER Dipped in Curry-sauce | 43 |
| 25. | TEMPEH in Onion Sauce | 44 |

Chapter 4 46
Low-fiber diet 46

26.	LOW-FIBER Omelet	46
27.	LOW-FIBER Tofu	47
28.	Low-fiber banana smoothie	48
29.	Homemade Apple-sauce	48
30.	Baked Salmon with Rosemary and Lemon	49
31.	Lemon Chicken Breasts	50
32.	Baked Spaghetti Squash with Parmesan Cheese	51
33.	Pork Chop	51
34.	Smoked Turkey-Wrapped Zucchini Sticks	52
35.	Balsamic Chicken, Tomatoes, and White Bean Salad	53
36.	CHICKEN Cacciatore	54
37.	CHICKEN Adobo	54
38.	Chicken and Bell Pepper Sauté	55
39.	CHICKEN Stir-fry	56
40.	ROSEMARY Chicken	57
41.	Turkey and Kale Sauté	57
42.	Turkey with Bell Peppers and Rosemary	58
43.	Easy Ground Turkey and Spinach Stir-Fry	59
44.	Rosemary Chicken Stew	60
45.	Same Miso Chicken	60
46.	Chicken Slow Cooker	61
47.	Chicken Thighs with Steamed Cauliflower	62
48.	Steamed Salmon with Lemon-Scented Zucchini	62
49.	Tomato Basil Omelet:	63
50.	Eggs with greens Nutritional values:	64
51.	White Bean Turkey Chili	65
52.	Orzo Chicken Salad with Avocado Lime Dressing	66
53.	CHICKEN Parmesan	67
54.	Buffalo Chicken	68
55.	Savory Waffles	69
56.	Mexican Morning Eggs	69

Chapter 5 70
Full Liquid Stage 70

57.	Banana Almond Milk Smoothie	70
58.	Raspberry Green Tea Smoothie	71
59.	Spinach and Berries Smoothie	71
60.	Cantaloupe Smoothie	72

61.	Tropical smoothie	72
62.	Blueberry smoothie	73
63.	Greens Smoothie	73
64.	Mixed Berry Smoothie	74
65.	Strawberry-Turmeric Smoothie	74
66.	Blueberry Chia Seed Smoothie	75
67.	Chocolate Cherry Shake	75
68.	Orange Apple Breakfast Shake	76
69.	Green Tea and Ginger Shake	76
70.	HOMEMADE Eggnog	77
71.	Homemade Vanilla Pudding	77
72.	COCONUT pudding	78
73.	Mango Pudding:	79
74.	ORANGE Pudding	79
75.	Homemade Pistachio Ice-cream	80
76.	Coconut milk ice-cream	80
77.	Banana Avocado Ice-cream	81
78.	Strawberry milk ice-cream	81
79.	Homemade mango ice cream	82
80.	Homemade Chocolate Ice Cream	82
81.	Homemade Vanilla Ice Cream	83
82.	PUMPKIN Soup	84
83.	SPINACH Soup	85
84.	TOMATO Soup	85
85.	KALE Soup	86
86.	Beans Soup	86
87.	CARROT Soup	87
88.	Mushroom and Ginger Soup	88

Chapter 6 .... **89**

Clear Liquid Stage **89**

89.	Bone Broth	89
90.	Chicken Broth	90
91.	Beef Broth	91
92.	Ginger-Mushroom Broth	92
93.	Chicken Wonton Broth:	92
94.	Chicken Consommé:	93
95.	Tomato Consommé:	94
96.	Vegetable Consommé	95
97.	Poached Black Sesame Salmon and Bok Choy Broth:	96
98.	Kanji	97
99.	Spicy Lemonade	97

100.	Ginger juice	98
101.	Fruit Punch	98
102.	Vegetable Juice	99
103.	Carrot and orange juice:	100
104.	Cranberry Juice	100
105.	White Grape Juice	101
106.	Pineapple juice	101
107.	Apple Juice	102
108.	Honey Lemon Tea	102
109.	Ginger Tea	103
110.	Iced Sweet Tea	103
111.	Cranberry iced green tea	104
112.	Black tea	105
113.	Spicy Milk Tea	105
114.	Turmeric Milk Tea	106

A 30 DAYS MEAL PLAN **107**
1ST 10 DAYS **107**
2ND 10 DAYS **107**
3RD 10 DAYS **107**
Conclusion **110**

Introduction

Diverticulitis is a form of colitis characterized by inflammation of the colon and is classified as an inflammatory bowel disease. If left unrecognized and untreated in a timely manner, the condition has the potential to escalate and require medical intervention in the form of surgery. According to the National Institute of Diabetes and Digestive and Kidney Diseases (NIDDK), the emergence of diverticulitis is attributed to the formation and subsequent inflammation or infection of diverticula, which are pouch-like structures that occur within the gastrointestinal tract. Diverticulitis is a prevalent form of diverticular disease. One of the most commonly observed presentations of diverticulitis is referred to as diverticulitis. Diverticulitis is a pathological condition characterized by the infection and inflammation of diverticula. The clinical presentation of diverticulitis is influenced by multiple factors, such as the specific location of the afflicted diverticulum, the severity of the inflammatory response, and the coexistence of other medical conditions. Diverticulitis may also arise due to various other underlying disorders. Approximately 70 percent of patients commonly experience discomfort in the lower left quadrant, rendering it the prevailing initial complaint. The sensation of discomfort is frequently characterized as crampy, and it is occasionally associated with alterations in an individual's customary bowel movement patterns. The presence of discomfort in the lower right quadrant of the abdomen may potentially indicate the manifestation of ascending colon disease, diverticulitis affecting the cecum on the right side, or a combination of both of these medical disorders. There is a possibility that this sensation of unease is being misconstrued as a case of acute appendicitis. In many clinical contexts, patients may exhibit symptoms such as fever or leukocytosis, which can arise due to a multitude of factors. There exists a certain level of symptom overlap between irritable bowel syndrome and moderate diverticulitis, thereby potentially causing confusion. Irritable bowel syndrome (IBS) is a gastrointestinal disorder that impacts the functioning of the digestive system. The etiology of diverticular infection and distension remains uncertain, despite several possibilities proposed by researchers and medical professionals. Conditions such as constipation and other gastrointestinal diseases have the potential to induce heightened intracolonic pressure, thereby increasing the likelihood of diverticular wall perforation, as supported by the prevailing hypothesis. Constipation is widely recognized as a prevalent etiological factor contributing to the development of diverticulitis. The presence of microorganisms or solid fecal matter within a diverticulum has the potential to cause both physical discomfort and, in certain instances, an infection. Despite the necessity of incorporating fiber-rich meals into one's diet, it is advisable to refrain from consuming such foods during an episode of diverticulitis due to their potential exacerbating effect on the condition. In the event that an individual experiences symptom such as fever, abdominal discomfort, vomiting, nausea, chills, constipation, or diarrhea, it is probable that they are experiencing a flare-up of diverticulitis. Nevertheless, in the event that an individual solely has symptoms of diarrhea or constipation, it is plausible to consider that diverticulitis may not be the underlying condition. It is advisable to schedule an appointment with the physician's office to commence treatment and obtain guidance regarding the use of a clear liquid diet. The clear liquid diet is a highly restrictive dietary regimen designed to promote relaxation and soothe the digestive tract. The dietary regimen exclusively consists of transparent fluids. A diverse range of liquids, including ice chips, water, fruit juices (without pulp), gelatin, ice pops (without pulp or fruit), tea, and coffee (without milk and cream), are deemed permissible. Once the signs of symptom alleviation become apparent, it is advisable to schedule a consultation with your main healthcare provider to deliberate on the feasibility of reintroducing a low-fiber diet. The determination of whether an individual can safely reintroduce low-fiber foods into their diet can be made by their primary care physician. In the initial stage, it is advisable to incorporate into one's diet fruits that have undergone cooking or canning processes, as well as soft vegetables devoid of their outer skins. Additionally, the consumption of fish, eggs, white bread, poultry, milk, low-fiber cereals, cheese, yoghurt, pasta, and rice is recommended. In addition, fruits that have undergone boiling or preservation in alcohol may also be consumed.

Chapter 1

Fundamentals Of Diverticulitis

What is Diverticulitis?

Diverticulitis is a chronic condition that impacts the digestive tract and is distinguished by the creation of pouches or sacs in the wall of the colon. This condition is also known as diverticulitis. This condition frequently causes a great deal of discomfort. There is the potential for both acute and chronic forms of diverticulitis. Diverticulitis is another name for the condition that is more generally referred to by its more popular name, diverticulosis. Diverticula is the term that is commonly used to refer to the pouches that are observed on the periphery of the longitudinal muscle that encases the intestinal wall. These pouches can be seen in people who have diverticulitis. Some people have pockets similar to these on their bodies. Diverticulitis is a condition that causes inflammation of the gut, and those who suffer from it are more likely to have diverticula than the general population. Diverticula are a type of structure that is located within the colon. No matter how old a person is, there is an extremely high probability that they have at least one of these pouches concealed on their person in some way. In most cases, the initial symptoms of this particular illness will show up in the colon or the big intestines. This is because the colon is the organ that processes food. Having said that, this isn't always going to be the case. On the other hand, the symptoms could show up in places other than the stomach as well. Nevertheless, for certain individuals, this sickness may also have an effect on the small intestine. Those who are getting on in years may find this to be particularly true. Something along these lines may happen. The inflammatory condition known as diverticulitis can present itself in a single diverticulum or in a large number of diverticula at the same time. This illness has the potential to impact the entire colon. Diverticula are pockets that can be found in the colon, and their medical term is diverticula. Diverticulitis is also known as diverticulitis. Diverticula can be found and identified if one is on the lookout for them. In addition, the manifestation of inflammation may take place at the same time as an acute infection, whose presence frequently has an adverse impact on the individual's overall state of health. Diverticulosis is a common medical condition that refers to the symptoms of diverticulitis that are not as severe as those of diverticulitis. The condition known as diverticulitis is a more serious form of diverticulosis. The condition can also worsen into diverticulitis, which is a more severe form of the condition. Inflammation of the diverticula is a hallmark of the more severe type of the disease, which is more commonly referred to as diverticulitis. A severe and lingering pain in the lower abdominal region is the clinical marker of diverticulitis that is observed the majority of the time in patients who have the disorder. Those who suffer from diverticulitis are diagnosed with the ailment. In certain extremely rare cases, in addition to the patient being in pain, they may also be exhibiting additional symptoms such as fever and confusion. These types of occurrences are quite unusual. This symptom is the one that is noted in clinical practice the great majority of the time. There is a possibility that the patient will experience a significant rise in the overall number of white blood cells that are already present in their blood. There is also a possibility that the patient will have a higher-than-normal level of white blood cells. In common parlance, the ailment known as diverticular disease is more commonly known as diverticulitis. Diverticular disease is a medical term. The formation of a number of tiny pouches within the lining of the intestines is one of the hallmark symptoms of the condition known as diverticulitis. These pouches get inflamed and transform into sacs as they progress. The phrase "diverticular disease" is used to refer to this condition. Diverticulitis is a term that is occasionally used to refer to the ailment that is more often known as diverticular disease. Diverticulitis occurs due to a number of different circumstances. The production of sacs that pierce the surface of the colon's outer layer and extend outward is what leads to the development of diverticula. Diverticulitis is a condition that can affect both children and adults. It is fair to refer to this particular ailment as a "silent killer" due to the fact that it has the capability of being misdiagnosed and untreated for a considerable amount of time. The disorder is referred to as a "silent killer" because of this reason. When the severity of the symptoms is minimal, there is a risk that this particular illness will go untreated, and it is possible that it will continue to be undiagnosed for a considerable amount of time before it is discovered. It is possible that the symptoms will present themselves as moderate digestive difficulties, such as light diarrhea or mild constipation. This is a possibility. On the other hand, it's always possible that the symptoms won't show up at all. On the other hand, there is also the possibility that none of these symptoms will manifest at all. There is a chance of this happening. Both of these scenarios have the potential to be misunderstood as falling within the limitations of what is considered to fall within the bounds of what is thought to fall within the limits of what is considered to fall within the bounds of what is seen to be regular or normal activity in the world of biology. The symptoms that were discussed before would gradually intensify until they revealed themselves as the first evidence that a flare was beginning to occur.

Juices can be consumed in their original state, but they do not include dietary fibre. On the other hand, it is strongly advised that before consumption, canned or frozen fruits and vegetables be peeled. This is because the peeling process removes harmful substances. Dried fruits, which include items like raisins, plums, apricots, and dates, are a crucial component of a diet that is high in both the quality and quantity of nutrients, as is general knowledge. Inexorably, in the same way that people do not always adhere to the same dietary patterns throughout the length of their life, the precise kinds of foods that are to be avoided in the context of diverticulitis will invariably differ from one instance of diverticulitis to the next. This is because people do not always adhere to the same dietary patterns throughout the course of their lives. The fundamental explanation for this phenomenon is that individuals do not always adhere to the same patterns of eating, which is why this phenomenon occurs. Our bad dietary patterns, our insufficient intake of critical nutrients, and the poisonous compounds that are created as a result of these behaviors are the key contributors to the problem that we are currently presented with. These are all factors that have led to the current state in which we find ourselves. All of these different aspects played a role in the development of the issue that we are currently facing. If you haven't already discovered this on your own, the present moment presents an excellent chance for you to cultivate an interest in the subject matter of health and nutrition. On the off chance that you have not already found this out on your own, I will tell you now.

After being aware of the detrimental impact that some foods have on one's health and well-being, it may be challenging for an individual to refrain from eating their preferred meals. This is especially true if the individual takes pleasure in the act of eating the foods in question. It is possible for us to have a feeling of emotional anguish when we restrict ourselves to our guilty pleasures, such as high-fat cheeseburgers, velvety chocolate, or even delicious bread. This is because when we deprive ourselves of these things, we are denying ourselves something that brings us pleasure. On the other hand, if one considers the situation from a more holistic point of view, it becomes abundantly evident that the vast majority of individuals put their future and their health ahead of the preferences they have for their own diet. Because particular foods have the potential to bring on uneasy feelings, it is common practice to keep a tight eye on how much of those foods are consumed.

This is done because those foods can create discomfort. The reason for this exercise is that particular meals have the potential to bring up uneasy sensations. Because of this, certain meals are avoided throughout this practice. People who struggle with recurring conditions like diverticulitis would benefit the most from this treatment because of its potential to prevent future episodes of such conditions. Diverticulitis is distinguished from other illnesses by the fact that inflammation or infection of the colon's microscopic pouches is its hallmark symptom. These pouches have the potential to become inflamed or infected if they become clogged with even the tiniest bits of undigested food or faeces. This is because even the smallest fragments of undigested food or faeces can cause inflammation and infection. One strategy to lessen the likelihood of developing diverticulitis is to steer clear of foods that are both high in fibre and high in the amount of water they contain. Nevertheless, there are dietary limits that are recommended to be adhered to, in addition to food choices that are encouraged, both during active episodes of diverticulitis and during periods of remission of the condition. These dietary restrictions and food choices may be found in both the Diverticulitis Diet and the Diverticulitis Diet for Active Diverticulitis.

The dietary restrictions and choices that were discussed earlier must, under all circumstances and at all times, be adhered to. It is recommended that a person who is experiencing symptoms that are symptomatic of diverticulitis, such as pain that is centered in the lower left side of the abdomen, fever, bloating, and diarrhoea, adhere to a liquid diet until the symptoms subside, or for the length of time that is indicated by a medical practitioner. Diverticulitis is an inflammation of the diverticulum, which is the tube that connects the large intestine to the small intestine. Maintaining the dietary routine that has been recommended is an absolute requirement if you want to decrease the severity of any future episodes of diverticulitis and possibly even stop them from occurring altogether. Antibiotics may offer momentary respite from excruciating pain and suffering; nevertheless, the use of these therapies for an extended period of time is associated with significant health risks that are comparable to those that are presented by the underlying illness. In addition, using antibiotics for an extended period of time might cause the body to become resistant to them, which reduces the antibiotics' efficacy. This happens when they are used for longer than the recommended time frame. When antibiotics are taken for an unusually long duration, this side effect is a distinct possibility. Because of this, it is frequently necessary to go through with a surgical operation that is potentially risky and invasive, which, in the end, causes a reduction in one's quality of life. Simply keep the term "itis" in your brain whenever you hear either of these names, and you will be able to tell them apart. This straightforward tactic is efficient and straightforward to use. When a patient is diagnosed with a medical disease that ends with the aforementioned word, the diagnosis nearly always signals that the patient is suffering from some type of inflammation in their body. When it comes to treating medical difficulties, one of the most popular techniques is to take precautions to limit the risk of the inflammation rupturing open. This is one of the most common approaches because it is so effective. In the event that the component is not functioning properly, there is a possibility that it will put the user's life in a situation of extreme danger.

The existence of perforations or a significant number of pouches is one of the most typical symptoms that a person has diverticulitis in their colon or large intestine, and it is also one of the most telling signals. Both the colon and the large intestine are potential sites of infection for diverticulitis. Despite the fact that they are referred to as "holes," these apertures are walled with a very thin layer of tissue that prevents waste and germs from accessing the inner surface of the colon. They are still dubbed "holes," but it doesn't stop them from doing this. These linings have what are colloquially known as "holes," but technically speaking, they are apertures. These apertures are found in the linings. The fragility of the lining, which makes it prone to tearing, renders it susceptible to rupturing when it is subjected to pressure that is above what is tolerable. This increases the likelihood of the lining tearing. As a consequence of this, the diverticulum will eventually become injured and will break apart. When this protective barrier is breached, bacteria and other potentially harmful substances are able to find their way onto the surface of the colon. This can eventually lead to a severe sickness if the barrier is not immediately restored, but it can also be avoided by repairing the barrier as soon as possible. This kind of damage has the potential to result in the development of a localized infection, the signs of which include the buildup of pus and germs in the affected area.

The presence of this infection allows for a diagnosis to be made. When the topic in question is brought up for discussion, the majority of the time, the condition in question is referred to as an abscess. The infection has a predisposition to spread beyond the confines of the colon wall, and it has the ability to have an effect on the organs that are placed nearby, such as the ovaries, the bladder, and the uterus. Additionally, the infection has a tendency to extend beyond the constraints of the colon wall. The production of fistulae in the bladder is a regular occurrence, and this phenomenon commonly leads to the development of holes in the bladder. Air passing through a patient's urinary tract when they are peeing is another common phenomenon that medical personnel observe in their patients. This takes place when the patient is voiding their bladder. It is a hard process since the treatment for the abscess includes the participation of other organs, each of which is vulnerable to the risk of being damaged. Diverticulitis, which is also referred to as diverticulosis, is an illness that is rather common and is defined by the absence of any visible symptoms. Diverticulosis is sometimes referred to as diverticulitis. The disease is defined by a pattern of symptoms that worsens over time, and there is now no medication that may halt or even reverse this progression of symptoms. The only way to exercise any kind of control over it is to discover any problems early on and take steps to avoid them from happening again by utilising preventative measures. This is the only way to exert any kind of control over it. A disease known as diverticulosis is characterized by the development of pouches in the colon that are not caused by cancer.

One of the risk factors for developing diverticulitis is heredity. The medical term for this ailment is diverticulosis. Diverticulitis is another name for it. Mycosis, also known as hypertrophy of muscle tissues, is the medical term for this ailment. The key reason for concern is the development of high-pressure zones as a direct result of mycosis, which is also known as the condition. The sigmoid colon, which may be found in the lower left quadrant of the abdominal region, is the site of the process that causes the colon to become denser and stiffer over time. This process takes place in the colon. In addition to an increase in the total number of muscle contractions, considerable constriction is a possibility among the symptoms of this condition. The growth of muscle is an effect that stems directly from this factor. As a consequence of these contractions, the patient will almost certainly be in a great deal of discomfort. These devices may also result in unusually increased pressures, which can lead to the pressurization of the walls of the colon, which can ultimately result in their rupture and infection within and around the colon wall. This can happen if the colon is pressurized to an abnormally high level. In addition, these devices have the potential to pressurize the colon, which can result in pressures that are far higher than normal. In addition to that, it's possible that these pressures are the outcome of the aforementioned technological devices. This is the condition that, in more severe cases, has the potential to lead to the development of diverticulitis. Maintaining a diet that is high in fibre and drinking a lot of fluids throughout the day are the two most important things that you can do in order to fully cure diverticulitis. The two things that will benefit you the most are these. It is entirely conceivable that by the time one has finished reading this cooking guide, they will have acquired the knowledge required to create great gourmet dishes that are characterized by the ease and speed with which they are created.

Additionally, one would have the ability to immediately limit the course of diverticulitis, a condition that either oneself or a member of one's family suffers from. This skill would be available 9k851to the individual immediately. After you have finished reading through this culinary encyclopedia, you will have the ability to take advantage of both of these chances. The cookbook provides a wide variety of culinary options that are appropriate for individuals who are looking for nutritional options that are low in residue, rich in fiber, and high in potassium. These possibilities are presented in the cookbook. Recipes for everything from breakfast to supper, with some snacks and drinks thrown in for good measure are included in this collection. Breakfast comes first in the day, followed by lunch, and then dinner is eaten at the end of the day.

What causes diverticulitis?

The precise factors that contribute to the development of diverticulitis remain a subject of ongoing discourse as researchers continue to discover and examine the underlying causes of this disease. Conversely, numerous investigations and rigorous analyses have demonstrated that the intake of a low-fiber diet may serve as the predominant factor contributing to the development of the disease. Conversely, in cases where the average dietary intake lacks enough fiber, the passage of stool may become challenging, necessitating increased exertion to promote its expulsion from the body. The term "constipation" is used to describe a commonly occurring medical problem. A dietary pattern characterized by insufficient fiber intake will lead to the formation of pouches. The application of pressure during defecation might result in heightened pressure within the colon, potentially causing the formation of diverticula within the colonic walls. The regions of the colon that exhibit inherent vulnerability are subjected to strain, resulting in the formation of small spherical structures that extend outward from the colon's surface. The excrement is momentarily stored at this particular site before its subsequent transfer to the subsequent pathway. The packets impede the whole passage of faces, resulting in the retention of a portion within their confines. Hence, the condition known as diverticulitis arises as a consequence of prolonged entrapment of fecal materials within the diverticula. The formation of growths and inflammation in the peri colonic region can be attributed to the multiplication of bacteria within the packets, as indicated by the findings of multiple studies. There exists a positive correlation between the prevalence of diverticulitis and regions characterized by insufficient dietary fiber content in their primary food sources. The prevalence of diverticulitis tends to increase with advancing age, although there is currently less empirical evidence to definitively support this observation. This phenomenon, however, is widely acknowledged and accepted, as it is a commonly held understanding that as individuals advance in age, their gut function tends to decline, thereby elevating their susceptibility to developing the aforementioned ailment.

Diverticulitis diet

Diverticulitis is a condition that can arise as a consequence of a diet lacking in dietary fiber. High-fat foods, such as red meat and heavily processed flours, have been implicated in the development of digestive disorders, specifically indigestion and constipation. In addition to the incorporation of a liquid-based dietary regimen, the consumption of a selection of low-fiber food items is also included in the prescribed diet. When identified in its early stages, the majority of instances of diverticulitis can be effectively treated by the implementation of a suitable dietary regimen and the administration of a select group of antibiotics. The recommended dietary approach for individuals with diverticulitis is the consumption of a low-fiber diet and increased fluid intake, with a special emphasis on beverages containing electrolytes. One of the crucial components in the management of diverticulitis involves the prevention of additional irritation to the intestines. One potential approach to facilitate the recuperation of the digestive tract following an episode of diverticulitis is the adoption of a bland diet, which often includes white rice, cooked poultry, mashed potatoes, and bananas. Consumption of fruits should be moderated, while dairy products should be restricted to modest servings of yogurt or kefir. Consumption of unprocessed fruits and vegetables has been found to be highly efficacious in the management of diverticulitis. These foods are rich in dietary fiber, a crucial component that aids in the management of this condition. Fruits and vegetables are considered significant contributors of dietary fiber due to their composition, which comprises both soluble and insoluble fiber. Soluble fiber exhibits the property of dissolution in water and undergoes fermentation within the colon. On the contrary, insoluble fiber exhibits limited solubility in water; however, it retains the capacity to absorb water, thereby undergoing softening to facilitate expeditious transit inside the gastrointestinal tract. Antibiotics are typically prescribed for the management of mild cases of diverticulitis, while individuals with severe diverticulitis may be advised to abstain from oral intake and adhere to a specialized dietary regimen until the cessation of bleeding and the alleviation of discomfort. The diverticulitis diet is widely advocated as an effective dietary approach for managing acute diverticulitis. While the intended duration of this dietary approach is limited, it can provide significant alleviation for people afflicted with diverticulitis. Additionally, it can be used by individuals with a susceptible gastrointestinal tract. The diverticulitis diet is primarily intended for individuals afflicted with diverticulitis; however, it can also provide advantages to individuals experiencing other forms of intestinal discomfort. Furthermore, people who are in good condition and desire to provide their digestive system with sufficient respite can derive advantages from adhering to this dietary regimen. It is advisable to refrain from the consumption of red and processed meat. The consumption of a diet that is rich in red and processed meats has the potential to elevate the likelihood of acquiring diverticulitis. Conversely, the consumption of a diet rich in vegetables, fruits, and whole grains has been linked to a decreased likelihood of developing certain health risks. In certain instances, individuals experiencing a diverticulitis flare may be advised to consume specific foods as well as implement dietary modifications to enhance tolerance of the illness and reduce the likelihood of exacerbation in the long term. It is often advised to adhere to a low-fiber diet until symptoms ameliorate, followed by a gradual transition to a high-fiber diet, in order to prevent recurrent exacerbations. Dietary fiber contributes to the softening and increased volume of fecal matter, facilitating its passage through the large intestine, also known as the colon. Furthermore, it has the effect of reducing pressure within the gastrointestinal system. The consumption of foods that are high in fiber has been shown to be beneficial in the management of symptoms associated with diverticulitis. Individuals who are below the age of 51, specifically women, are advised to consume a daily intake of 25 grams of dietary fiber, while males in the same age group are recommended to have 38 grams of dietary fiber each day. Individuals who are 51 years of age or older, specifically women and men, are recommended to consume 21 grams and 30 grams of dietary fiber per day, respectively.

Chapter 2

Introduction To Diverticulitis

Four stages comprise the diverticulitis diet: the maintenance stage, the clear liquid stage, the complete liquid stage, and the low-fiber stage. Each of these plays a unique role in the facilitation of recovery from diverticulitis flare-ups and the prevention of diverticulitis flare-ups in the future. In addition, each of these factors contributes to the prevention of future diverticulitis flare-ups.

The Clear Liquid Stage

At this point in the progression of the diverticulitis, it is essential to refrain from consuming anything other than what are known as "clear liquids." These are essentially nutritional drinks; when they are at room temperature, they are liquid and translucent, and their composition does not include any solid components. Although it could look as though this does not provide enough nutrition, the fact is quite the opposite: broths, juices, teas, and gelatin might all supply you with enough nutrients to last you through the day. This stage normally lasts between two and three days, the length of time it occupies being determined by the point at which the individual thinks that a significant improvement has occurred in the severity of their symptoms. When brought to room temperature, most transparent liquids exhibit the behaviour of fluids; however, there are a few significant exceptions to this rule. In most situations, they do not include a wide variety of nutrients in the appropriate amounts. The vast majority of the time, they possess the property of translucence. Clear liquids include things like water, plain gelatin, chicken broth, bone broth, vegetable broth, and the majority of forms of tea that do not contain any additional milk or cream.

Vegetable broth is also an example of a clear liquid. If you are trying to determine whether or not anything is a clear liquid, the most crucial thing to check for is whether or not the product contains any kind of milk or cream in any form. If it does, then you can safely assume that the product does not qualify as a clear liquid. It is not commonly believed to be a heavy liquid, and there is no type of solid mass floating around in the mixture where it is being held. Assuming that it is capable of meeting these requirements, the liquid in question ought to be see-through. During the time that you are on the clear liquid diet, it is absolutely necessary for you to abstain from drinking anything that does not satisfy any of the requirements that were discussed earlier in this section. This pertains to both solid and liquid items. Because of this, the diet will have the opposite effect of what you were expecting it to, and you will have to start over from the very first day. You should refrain from consuming anything that is solid, as well as anything that contains milk or cream (or any other form of dense dairy product, such as cheese or yoghurt). Consuming drinks that are clear has two purposes: first, it gives your digestive tract a chance to relax, and second, it makes the diverticulitis symptoms that you're feeling less severe. Both of these benefits can be realized by drinking more clear liquids. This is the very first step in the process, and as such, it is of the utmost significance to both the recovery from diverticulitis and the prevention of flare-ups. This is the step that paves the way for all of the other phases, and as a direct result of this, it is also the step that the majority of individuals will find to be the most challenging to stick to. However, this phase only lasts for a few days (or until the symptoms begin to lessen), so as long as you are able to stick with it for the short duration that it lasts, you will be able to fulfil the goals that you have set for yourself and achieve success in the process. A day spent adhering to a diet of clear liquids is not very taxing on the willpower. For breakfast, one could, for instance, decide to create chicken broth to go along with their iced tea, and they might also want to serve gelatin on the side. My option for lunch was a bowl of tomato consommé accompanied by fruit punch. You do not need to be concerned because the odorless liquid is not nearly as harmful as it may sound, despite the fact that its description makes it sound like it would be an unpleasant experience. Even if it proves to be difficult, it will only persist for a few days, so there is not much need to be concerned about it at this point.

The full liquid stages

The stage known as "full liquid" refers to the consumption of liquids that are in their whole form. This stage represents a progression beyond the clear liquid phase. During the phase characterized by full liquid intake, it is imperative to bear in mind that all items previously specified as permissible during the clear liquid stage remain suitable for consumption. Individuals will not be restricted to the use of solely complete liquids, but rather they will be advised to avoid any substances that are denser than full liquids, including solid foods. The complete liquid phase involves gradually raising the temperature of the intestines to facilitate food digestion while minimizing the exacerbation of diverticulitis symptoms. The aforementioned process was initiated by the initial phase, characterized by a transparent liquid, and it is anticipated that the subsequent phase, known as the complete liquid stage, will further advance this process. One may inquire, as any individual would in a typical scenario, about the precise definition of full liquids. Similar to clear liquids, complete liquids typically exist in a liquid state at room temperature or, alternatively, transition into a liquid state at room temperature. Nevertheless, the majority of dairy products are encompassed, with cheese being the sole exception. For example, a comprehensive liquid diet allows for the consumption of thin, creamy soups, milk, ice cream, milkshakes, various puddings and custards, as well as Jello. It is crucial to adhere to a dietary restriction of consuming only full liquids during this stage, as consuming anything heavier would undermine the intended goal of the full liquid stage. If one is uncertain about the classification of a substance as a complete liquid, it is advisable to refer to online resources prior to consuming it. Prohibited activities during the full liquid stage can be readily discerned in a broad sense. Selecting food items that possess a solid state and lack the ability to undergo melting is evidently an unfavorable choice. It is sometimes assumed that cheese is an allowable component of a full liquid diet due to the prevalence of dairy products in such diets. However, this assumption is incorrect. Cheese is classified as a solid food, and as a result, it is subject to prohibition. In a manner akin to the clear liquid diet, soups containing solid dietary components such as potatoes or meat are likewise prohibited. Eggs can be included in a full liquid diet, provided that they undergo thorough pasteurization. If this appears to be unfavorable, there is no need for concern. I am prepared to assist you. One item that is permissible for consumption on a full liquid diet is eggnog, and this book provides a recipe for its preparation. Once again, the objective of the full liquid stage aligns with that of the clear liquid stage. To be more precise, it represents a progression from the preceding phase, characterized by the presence of a transparent fluid. The primary objective of both of these dietary approaches is to provide respite to the digestive tract, thereby preparing it for the two preventive phases of the diverticulitis diet. The individual has already provided their digestive system with respite by adhering to a diet consisting solely of transparent fluids. Consequently, it is now appropriate to gradually introduce things that require greater digestive effort. This process facilitates the gradual adaptation of the gastrointestinal system to increasingly challenging dietary components, thereby enabling the use of preventive measures (such as low-fiber and maintenance stages) to mitigate the risk of recurrent diverticulitis episodes. One additional similarity between the full liquid stage and the clear liquid stage is the predominant consumption of liquid-based substances. As an illustration, an individual adhering to a full liquid diet may commence their day by consuming cream of wheat, a recipe for which is also included inside this publication, accompanied by a serving of fruit punch. It is evident that the complete liquid phase is characterized by a lesser degree of restriction in comparison to the clear liquid phase. The trend of decreasing limitations will persist as one progresses through the text.

The low-fiber stage

You are now at the point where you can return to consuming solid foods. Consuming foods that, as the name suggests, are low in fiber is the focus of the low-fiber stage of the diet. This stage also indicates the transition into the prevention stages, which are aimed more toward the prevention of future diverticulitis outbreaks than the recovery from previous flare-ups. This stage also marks the transition into the prevention stages. Along with the maintenance stage, which will be discussed in more detail in just a moment, the low-fiber stage will ensure that your intestines are ready for everything you may throw at them. This diet contains very little fiber, so following it should result in few and infrequent bowel movements, thereby reducing the likelihood of a subsequent outbreak. In a general sense, the foods that you consume during this time should not have a lot of fiber in any form. You are allowed to consume foods that are low in fiber throughout this stage of the diet. These items include chicken and other types of poultry, eggs, fish, lean meats, and solid dairy foods (even cheese!). Be aware, however, that there is a possibility that some of the recipes from the clear liquid or full liquid stages will not be suitable for the low-fiber stage. If you intend to use any of those recipes for the low-fiber stage, you should research the internet to determine whether or not any of the Ingredients contain excessive amounts of fiber.

In general, you should make sure that the food you are consuming has a fiber content that is lower than 3 grams per serving. This will help you maintain a healthy digestive system. At this point in the process, you should avoid eating foods that have a high fiber content because these will slow down your digestion. Wild rice, avocados, items made with whole wheat grain, the vast majority of nuts and/or seeds, uncooked versions of vegetables and fruits (such as corn and berries), and other foods that are high in fiber should be avoided at all costs. As was the case with the stages that came before it, the eating of any of these categories of foods will render this stage's preventative benefits ineffective. Again, if you are uncertain about the fiber content of a particular item, it is smart to confirm its fiber content using the internet. The recipes in the low-fiber area are all guaranteed to be low in fiber, of course, but if you are uncertain about the fiber content of a single ingredient, it is guaranteed to be low in fiber. Consuming meals that are low in fiber content serves no purpose other than to make digestion simpler, as this is not the reason for doing so. They do not encourage the formation of stools as much as their alternatives that are high in fiber, which means that they are far less likely to induce flare-ups in the symptoms that you experience as a result of your diverticulitis. This assures that you will have not only made a major impact on the symptoms of the flare-up in your diverticulitis that inspired you to start this diet, but that you will also have contributed to the prevention of the worsening of diverticulitis symptoms in the future. The flare-up in your diverticulitis was what prompted you to start this diet. You will observe that a day that occurs during the low-fiber stage does not seem to be as difficult as a day that occurs during the full liquid stage or the clear liquid stage. For breakfast each morning, you will most likely be served something that is comparable to pancakes or grits prepared in a Southern way. You may eat chicken roasted with lemon and rosemary for lunch. The chicken would be delicious. You could cook yourself a meal consisting of homemade lasagna made from scratch for dinner. You can find a recipe for each of the meals I just mentioned in the section dedicated to foods low in fiber, so go ahead and indulge.

The maintenance stage

In the maintenance stage of the diverticulitis diet, the focus is squarely on achieving the greatest possible reduction in inflammatory symptoms.

When compared to the nutritional options accessible during previous stages, the ones that are offered throughout the final stage are significantly laxer. At this point in the process, the primary concentration is placed on the consumption of foods that are either anti-inflammatory or, at the very least, do not have an intrinsically inflammatory nature. These sorts of dietary decisions are often recognized as acceptable. This book includes a compilation of twenty different recipes that have been developed specifically for the maintenance stage. In addition to facilitating the development of new knowledge and abilities, the dining experience provided at each meal is one that is both pleasurable and interesting. It would be helpful if you could look through all of the items in the table of contents to figure out which topics are most interesting to you. Please feel free to do so. As was said before, the consumable things that are considered to be within acceptable parameters include any and all chemicals that have anti-inflammatory qualities. Alternatively, this applies to anything that does not directly cause inflammation in the body. It is recommended that you give anti-inflammatory foods higher priority in your diet in order to achieve the best possible results from your food choices. You will, nevertheless, be able to keep your state of well-being at a satisfactory level so long as you abstain from consuming things that encourage inflammation. It has been shown that certain foods contain qualities that can reduce inflammation in the body. These consist of foods like avocados and potatoes that are high in beneficial fats and are classified as fruits and vegetables. In addition, seeds and nuts, as well as some types of seafood that are high in omega-3 fatty acids, have been linked to a reduction in inflammation. Particularly notable for its beneficial properties is the use of turmeric powder, which can be found in a wide variety of anti-inflammatory recipes due to its widespread application. Foods that have been subjected to a high level of processing, foods that contain red meat, and foods that contain refined carbohydrates are not advised for ingestion. These kinds of remarks are notorious for the fact that they are highly provocative, and you should make a point to steer clear of them under any and all circumstances. The primary goal of the maintenance stage is to assist in the continuous avoidance of diverticulitis flare-ups. This is the primary objective of the maintenance stage.

The inflammation of the gastrointestinal tract is the primary contributor to the development of diverticulitis. This inflammation makes it easier for bacteria to colonise the diverticula, which in turn can lead to infection. As a result, treating this inflammatory illness will also reduce the risk of diverticulitis developing in the digestive tract. The maintenance stage is believed to be the most lenient of the four stages, as it enables the intake of a wide variety of meals. Many people view this phase as the most lenient. When deciding what to eat for breakfast, some people choose to limit their options to foods that do not cause inflammation. This is something that they may do if they want to. This way of eating permits the consumption of a wider variety of dishes, such as scrambled eggs or a frittata prepared with mushrooms and kale. This is because the diet allows for the intake of a wider range of foods. Now that you have an understanding of the four stages of the diverticulitis diet, you are in a position to begin working toward curing your diverticulitis and regaining your health. The following is an exhaustive compilation of sixty mouthwatering foods that are appropriate for all of the aforementioned levels. I have faith that participating in this activity will be enjoyable for you.

Chapter 3
Maintenance stage
1. Delicious Oatmeal with Turmeric Powder

Oatmeal is widely regarded as a highly favorable food choice, leaving little room for debate. Nevertheless, the utilization of anti-inflammatory oatmeal is deemed more

advantageous, and it is precisely this particular recipe that we shall proceed to prepare. This particular culinary formula, which incorporates the inclusion of turmeric powder, is designed to produce a quantity sufficient to serve two individuals.

Ingredients:

- Two splashes of milk
- The suggested quantity is one teaspoon of turmeric powder.
- Two cups of water.
- One unit of measurement consisting of a volume of rolled, whole oats, equivalent to approximately 237 milliliters.

Direction:

- Put the oats into a wide pot containing two cups of vigorously boiling water. Reduce the flame to a moderate setting and proceed to cook for a duration of ten minutes, ensuring to stir the mixture at regular intervals.
- Incorporate approximately equal proportions of milk and turmeric powder into the mixture after approximately five minutes, while maintaining a consistent

stirring motion. After the completion of the cooking process for the oatmeal, transfer it into a suitable receptacle and proceed to select from a diverse range of potential toppings. Alternatively, it is possible to consume it in its unadorned

state.

- Regardless of the perspective, this oatmeal possesses both nutritional value and a pleasing taste.

2. Banana and Almond Butter Oatmeal

favorable food choice, leaving little room for debate. This particular oatmeal consists of banana and almond butter is really good for guy health.

Nutritional values:

- 6 g Fat
- 8 g Protein
- 66 g Carbohydrate
- Calorie count:375

Ingredients:

- Almond milk
- Almond butter
- Oats
- Bananas
- Honey

Process:

• Start by combining almond milk and oats in a pot. Cook on low flame until almost all liquid has evaporated from the pan.

• Then, after the mixture has reached the right consistency, add the remaining banana slices and almond butter.

• Please switch off the stove. Put the muesli to a designated receptacle for presentation purposes. Banana slices should be stacked and served with honey on top. The honey's nutritional value is left out. If you're having trouble getting enough protein to meet your macros, try adding a scoop or half a scoop of whey protein.

3. Home Brewed Red Wine

In accordance with my authority, I hereby proclaim this publication to be a cookbook intended for those of advanced age and maturity. Therefore, this recipe will outline the process of producing homemade red wine. The outcome will yield a product that is abundant in taste and offer a straightforward set of instructions to adhere to. This recipe will produce a quantity of one gallon of flavorful red wine.

Ingredients:

- A total volume of eight cups of fresh water.
- A quantity of five pounds of red grapes that have been washed.
- A quantity of two pounds of granulated sugar. One unit of wine yeast.

- One unit of wine yeast.

Direction:

- In the designated vessel for the fermentation process, position the 5-pound quantity of grapes at the base and afterwards crush them into a pulpy consistency. In a distinct vessel, fully dissolve the entirety of the sugar within the water, then incorporating this sugar-water solution into the receptacle containing the grapes.

- Firstly, proceed by heating 3 ounces of water to a temperature that is comfortably lukewarm. Subsequently, pour the contents of the wine yeast packet into the water. Please refrain from agitating this combination. Allow the

substance to remain undisturbed for a duration of approximately 15 minutes. After a duration of 15 minutes, gently agitate the combination in order to uniformly disperse the yeast particles inside the water, subsequently introducing this amalgamation into the vessel containing the water and grapes.

- Presently, it is possible to combine several elements. Gently agitate the

Ingredients within the fermentation container through stirring or shaking. Allow the container to be placed in a location with a warm temperature, ensuring that it does not exceed 80 degrees Fahrenheit, for a duration of around seven days.

Agitate the solution on two occasions within a 24-HOUR period. Following a period of seven days, it is advised to transfer the fluid into a separate receptacle, taking caution to avoid any disruption to the sediment layer situated at the lowermost part.

- Acquire saran wrap and a rubber band. Position the saran wrap atop the aperture of the subsequent receptacle, and secure it firmly by affixing a rubber band around the periphery of the orifice. In the event that your fermentation container possesses an airtight lid, it is advisable to refrain from securely affixing the lid onto the container. The saran wrap functions as an airlock, facilitating the release of gases produced by the yeast while preventing the re-entry of air. It is

recommended to let this to remain undisturbed for a duration of four weeks.

- After the fermentation process has ceased, proceed to transfer the liquid into bottles. The concept of age as a desired attribute.

4. Ginger Carrot Soup with Turmeric Powder

The provided recipe provides a quantity of ginger carrot soup with turmeric powder sufficient to serve three individuals.

Ingredients:

- Ginger Salt
- Black pepper
- Carrots, chopped and peeled Vegetable stock
- Shallots
- Garlic clove
- Olive oil, extra-virgin
- Orange-juice and orange-zest Turmeric powder

Direction:

- Acquire a sizable saucepan and place it atop a stovetop burner set to moderate flame. Incorporate the shallots and olive oil into the mixture. Proceed to cook for a duration of 5 minutes.

- Subsequently, incorporate the turmeric powder, ginger, orange zest, garlic, pepper, and salt, and thoroughly combine the Ingredients. Allow this mixture to simmer for a duration of two minutes. Following a two-minute interval, introduce the carrots into the frying process and proceed to cook them for an additional three minutes. Initially, commence the process by bringing the orange juice and vegetable stock to a state of boiling. Subsequently, proceed to decrease the flame to a level conducive for simmering. Maintain the current temperature for a duration of twenty-five minutes.

- To purée the soup, it is recommended to use a blender that is capable of effectively ventilating steam, and to do it in batches. It is imperative to verify that the blender possesses the capacity to effectively dissipate steam, as failure to do so may result in an accumulation of pressure within the apparatus, ultimately leading to the expulsion of the lid and the dispersion of scalding hot soup in all directions.

- The dish should be served while hot in order to fully appreciate its flavors.

5. Ginger Soya-milk Soup

This is a very interesting flavorful dish. Traditionally dairy based milk is used for this. But the soya milk version is tastier and healthier for diverticulitis patients.

Ingredients:

- plain unsweetened vegan milk
- ginger powder
- salt
- red chile powder or cayenne
- water
- cilantro

Method:

- On medium-high heat, in a pot, slightly boil the soy milk
- Put salt along with spices like red chile powder, green thai chilies, and water in addition to the ginger powder. Add the cilantro and simmer until thickened and then serve the dish with naan.

6. Anti-Inflammatory Stir-fry

The following recipe provides instructions for preparing a flavorful stir-fry with a spicy kick, known for its potential anti-inflammatory properties. The given measurements are intended to create two servings.

Ingredients:

- A pinch of ground black pepper
- One-half cup of tomato paste
- one-tenth of a teaspoon of ground turmeric
- Gluten-free chicken sausage in four links. Three garlic cloves, minced
- One bag of "Healthy 8 Veggie Mix." Those are available at Trader Joe's.
- 1 tsp. of virgin coconut oil

Direction:

- Place a frying pan on a stovetop burner set to medium heat, and proceed to heat the coconut oil until it reaches a liquid state. Mince the garlic cloves and include them into the pan, allowing them to cook for a duration of one minute.

•Subsequently, incorporate the constituents of the Healthy 8 Veggie Mix, succeeded by the inclusion of turmeric powder and black pepper. The chicken sausage should be diced into small pieces and incorporated into the skilletsubsequent to the vegetables being cooked for a duration of five minutes.Combine the components of this combination thoroughly and let it simmer for an extra duration of two minutes.

•Finally, incorporate the tomato sauce into the mixture, reduce the heat, and let it simmer for an extra duration of two minutes. Present the food on a plate or

within a bowl, then partake in its consumption.

7. Salad with Kale, Onions, and Apple Cider Vinegar

You won't be able to adequately convey how good this salad is to others if you make it using the following recipe, which calls for kale, onions, and apple cider vinegar. Thisdish will appeal most to vegetarians and those individuals who value vegetables above meat as their primary protein source. After completing all of the steps in this recipe, you will have a total quantity of 2 cups.

Ingredients:
- chopped kale
- Chopped onion
- kosher salt
- apple cider vinegar
- water
- Extra-virgin olive oil

Direction:

- To get started, grab a flat surface pot and put it in the oven on the rack that isdirectly in the center. The onion should be added first, followed by the salt, andthen the oil should be drizzled on top. Stir it at sporadic intervals over the course of the next three to five minutes as it cooks. Once the kale has been included, give the mixture a good toss. Include the two tablespoons of water in the very last step of the process. A further two minutes of cooking time should be allotted after the lid of the pan has been placed back on it. After the first two minutes, after which you should add an extra two tablespoons of water, proceed to continue cooking for the subsequent four minutes.

- After all of this has been completed, take off the lid of the pan, then slowly pour in the vinegar while swirling the mixture. Enjoy yourselves!

8. Cucumber and Smoked-Salmon Lettuce Wraps

This recipe is light, healthy and delicious and it can be eaten as an easy breakfast or snack option. The given measurements are intended to create four servings.

Ingredients:

- Lettuce leaves (8)
- English cucumber (½)
- Smoked salmon (8 ounces)
- Fresh chives
- Caesar Salad Dressing

Direction:

- On a dish, place your lettuce leaves.
- Equal distribute cucumber slices among your lettuce leaves.
- Top each leaf with the smoked salmon.
- Garnish with chives & drizzle each wrap with the Salad

9. Flax-Almond Porridge

This delicious bowl of porridge recipe is a good breakfast option and can be used for four servings.

Ingredients:

- Bananas
- Almond milk (2 cups)
- Raw honey
- Almond meal (3/4 cup)
- Flax meal
- Ground cinnamon
- Maple syrup
- Apple

Direction:

- Place your saucepan over the medium heat.
- Add & stir together flax meal, almond meal, honey, almond milk, & bananas until smooth.
- Sprinkle your cinnamon over the mixture.

- Simmer for around 3-4 minutes.
- Pour this porridge into the bowls.
- Add apples over the top.
- Serve it.
- Enjoy!

10. Blueberry-Millet Breakfast Bake

This delicious recipe is a good breakfast option and can be used for four servings.

Ingredients:
- Millet (2 cups)
- Blueberries (2 cups)
- Applesauce ((2 cups)
- Coconut oil (⅓ cup)
- Fresh ginger
- Ground cinnamon

Direction:
- Preheat your oven to 350°F.
- Drain & rinse your millet for around 1-2 minutes.
- Transfer it to your large bowl.
- Gently fold in your blueberries, coconut oil, applesauce, ginger, & cinnamon.
- Cover with aluminum foil.
- Place your dish into the preheated oven.
- Bake them for around 40 minutes.
- Then, remove your foil & then, bake them for almost 15 minutes more.

11. Applesauce Burger with Spinach Salad

This delicious and healthy burger recipe can be used for four servings

Ingredients:
- Chopped jalapeno (1 pc.)
- Mashed cumin (2 tsp.)
- Diced garlic (2 tsp.)
- Crushed dark beans (2 14.5 oz. jars)

- Raw yam (2 cups)
- Beaten egg (1 pc.)
- Plain breadcrumbs (1 cup)
- Whole wheat burger buns

Direction:

- Preheat the grill.
- Combine as one the egg whites, cereal, onions. Furthermore, ¼ cup fruit purée. Add the chicken. Blend everything well and make a burger patty.
- Shower non-stick covering on oven skillet. Put the burger on the rack and cook for around 5 minutes prior to turning over. Sear for an additional 5 minutes or on the other hand until the meat is at this point not pinkish in shading.
- Heat the remainder of the fruit purée and pour over the burger. (Test with the measures of fruit purée and cereal until your scope the ideal consistency.)
- While the burger is as yet cooking, whisk together some dressing fixings for certain pounded strawberries.
- Get a plate of mixed greens bowl and blend the tomato, onion, and strawberries together. Shower with dressing. Serve.

12. Blackened Chicken Avocado Power Bowl

Nutritional values:
- 57 g Protein
- 30 g Fat
- 28 g Carbohydrate
- Calorie COUNT:602

Ingredients:
- Powdered Chilli
- Powdered Garlic
- Powdered Onion
- Cumin
- Chicken breast
- Broccoli florets
- Yellow Bell paper
- Olives

- Chickpeas
- Red Cabbage
- Avocado
- Italian seasoning

Process:

- In the beginning, rub the chicken with the spices. Chili powder, onion powder, garlic powder, salt, paprika, cumin, Italian seasoning, and pepper should all be mixed together in a bowl for this.
- To season the chicken, sprinkle some of the spice blend on top and rub it in. In a heavy-bottomed pan set over a moderate flame, add a third of the oil.
- Cook the chicken for a few minutes on each side in a pan with heated oil. Third, roast the veggies in an oven. Prepare a 425 F oven.
- Spread the bell peppers, broccoli and chickpeas out on a pan for baking. Before tossing the veggies, add the rest of the oil. Toss with salt, pepper, and a pinch of the spice blend. Gently toss. Disperse it uniformly.
- Insert the baking parchment into the oven and subject it to a temperature of 400°F for the purpose of baking. The baking process should be continued for a duration of fifteen minutes, or until such time that the veggies have reached a state of tenderness. To serve, combine the avocado and red cabbage with theroasted vegetables. Sprinkle with chicken and serve.

13. Brown Rice Bowl with Turkey

Ingredients:

- Brown rice
- Chicken broth
- Soya sauce
- Olive oil
- Scallions
- Sesame seeds
- Salt
- Pepper
- Turkey breast
- Baby spinach
- Sesame oil

Method:

- In order to prepare rice, warm up a pan of suitable size over a moderate flame. Put in 14 cups of water, 12 cups of broth, some salt, and the rice. Make sure to put a lid on it.

- When the water in the pot begins to boil, reduce the heat. Allow the rice to

simmer until it is cooked. Add additional liquid at this time if necessary. Make sure your oven is preheated at 425 degrees F.

- Use foil to line a baking pan. To cook, spritz the food.

- The turkey should be flavored with a combination of salt and pepper and leave it where it is on the baking sheet. Coat the turkey with half of the soy sauce. Set the oven timer for thirty to forty five minutes, or until the food has been perfectly

browned, and then place the baking sheet inside. After 20 minutes in the oven, flip the turkey breast over. A meat thermometer inserted into the center of a cooked turkey should read at least 165 degrees Fahrenheit.

- To chop the turkey, number seven is to take it out of the oven. Use aluminum foil to cover it, but only loosely. Wait 5 minutes and then try again. The turkey should be sliced very thinly. 8 Put the remaining soy sauce, the scallions, and the spinach into the rice. Turn the heat up and add the rest of the stock to the rice. Maintain a healthy blend. 9 - Dish up a bowl of rice. Throw some turkey on there and call it a day.

- To serve, drizzle with sesame oil and sprinkle with sesame seeds.

14. Spiced Mango Soup with Tofu

This simple and delicious dish has a unique sweet, tangy and spicy flavor.As it has turmeric it is also anti-inflammatory.

Ingredients:

TOFU:

- firm tofu
- Vegetable oil
- Chili powder
- cinnamon powder
- Himalayan pink salt
- Mixed herbs
- Turmeric powder
- Shallots
- ginger

- cloves of garlic
- water
- Any vegan oil
- cumin seeds
- 2 bay leaves
- Canned coconut milk
- Unsweetened ripe mango pulp or puree
- salt
- vinegar
- black pepper
- Indian spice blend
- chopped cilantro

Method:

Tofu: Cut the thick tofu slab into pieces. They must be placed on a fresh dish towel. Place a second dish towel on top. Wait ten minutes after placing a weight of about 10 pounds on top. Additionally, pressured tofu is an option. Slices of tofu should be chopped into cubes.

- Put some oil in a cast-iron and heat it over a moderate flame. When using heated oil, tilting the pan ensures even coverage. Stir continuously after adding the tofu and sauté for 4 minutes, or until the sides are lightly browned. Salt is added, andthe chili powder, cinnamon, garammasala, and salt are mixed together thoroughly. After 2 more minutes, take it off the hob.

- To make the thick soup, put the shallots, garlic, and ginger in a blender with two cups of water and purée until completely smooth. In a large cast-iron heat, the oil over moderate temperature. After the oil has heated, add the cloves, bay leaves, and ground cumin seeds. The wait will just be a minute. When the onion mixture has started to dry and lost its raw aroma, stir in the onion puree. To prevent sticking, stir often during the first 13-15 minutes. Mix the turmeric,cider, salt, and mango flesh into the coconut cream thoroughly. Move the tofu and the rest of the Ingredients from the tofu pan into the cast-iron pot. Toss some black pepper.

- Combine everything, lid the pan, and simmer it until the sauce boils. Lower the flame and simmer the sauce,put the lid on until the desired consistency is reached. To your liking, adjust the salt and tang. Try adding another half teaspoon of sugar if the mango pulp isn't sweet enough. Garam masala and cilantro should be used as a garnish and served hot.

15. Garlic Butter Chicken Meatballs with Cauliflower Rice

Nutritional value:
- Calorie COUNT:342

Ingredients:
- Turkey or chicken
- Garlic
- Paper flakes
- Chicken stock
- Parsley or cilantro
- Hot sauce
- Cheese
- Italian seasoning
- Butter
- crumbled bouillon cube
- Cauliflower
- Salt
- Paper

Process:
- In a microwave-safe bowl, place the cauliflower rice. The rice should be covered with water and the lid placed on it. Prepare for roughly 2 minutes on high heat. Verify that the cauliflower rice is ready to be served. Added seconds of cooking time may be necessary.

- To make meatballs in a bowl, combine the ground chicken with the garlic,bouillon cube, half of the parsley, cheese, Italian seasoning, red pepper flakes, and cracked pepper. Form the Ingredients into meatballs and set them aside on a platter. Third, melt half the butter in a cast-iron pot set over low flame. Once the meatballs have browned on all sides and absorbed all of the pink, remove them from the pan. While the meatballs are in the oven, use a slotted spoon to sprinkle them with the cooking juices. Take the meatballs and put them on a platter to set aside.

- Put the rest of the butter into the pan. Stir in the remaining parsley, hot sauce,red pepper flakes, minced garlic, and hot sauce once the butter has melted. Bake it for a little while. Turn off the heat and to taste, add pepper and a pinch of salt to the food. Serving suggestion

- Fill a bowl with cauliflower rice. Toss meatballs with cauliflower rice and serve. The meatballs and cauliflower rice are ready to be served, so pour the sauce over the top.

- Cauliflower rice is optional; ordinary rice works just as well. Due to the switch to the healthier alternative of cauliflower rice, the dietary values will shift. Seven,you can prepare the chicken, rice, and sauce in advance and store them in individual meal containers in the fridge.
- Microwave to reheat and serve.

16. Lentil Garbanzo Soup with Turmeric

Lentil soup is a comfort food. Both protein and carbs are abundant in it. It also has turmeric powder which has anti-inflammatory properties.

Ingredients:

- Sliced onions (2 laptops.)
- Sliced celery (1 cup)
- Chopped carrots (1 cup)
- Mashed ginger (2 tsp.)
- Minced garlic (1 tsp.)
- Turmeric (1 tsp.)
- Ground cumin (1/2 tsp.)
- Ground cayenne pepper (1/4 tsp.)
- Vegetable stock or stock (6 cups)
- Lentils (1 cup)
- Undrained dainty diced tomatoes (1 14.5-OZ. can)

Direction:

- Sauté onions in a huge pot over medium to high flame for 3 - 4 minutes or until onions are delicate.
- Add celery and carrots into the pot and continue to cook for an extra five minutes. Mix in garlic, garam masala, turmeric, cumin and cayenne pepper into the pot and continue to cook for 30 additional seconds.
- Add the cups of stock, lentils, garbanzo beans and tomatoes into the pot, then, at that point, continue to mix the fixings until every one of them are joined.
- Cook the stock for an hour and a half or until the lentils are delicate.
- For a creamier and thicker soup, you can take out a portion of the stock, puree it with a food processor, then, at that point, set it back into the pot and mix.

17. SPLIT Pea Soup with Spices and Coconut Ingredients::

Ingredients:

- chickpeas (chana dal)
- water
- Ginger paste
- Spicy sauce
- Vegan masala
- Garam masala
- Olive or plant oil
- Butter
- Fresh Cheese
- cilantro
- Chaat Masala, for garnish
- frozen green peas, thawed if frozen
- Cilantro, lemon juice, chopped onion, for garnish Dinner rolls
- pepper flakes, for garnish

Method:

- Split peas (Dal): Put 3 1/2 cups water, turmeric, and the spice into a saucepan. Split peas need 30–40 minutes of cooking time in a partially covered pot over medium heat, or until extremely soft. Add the salt and sugar and mix well. While you prepare the tempering, turn the heat down to a simmer.

- Tempering A small skillet with oil in it should be heated over medium heat. It takes just about a minute for the coconut flakes to get brown in the oven. Put the coconut flakes in a bowl and remove them from the heat. For one minute, or until aromatic, heat oil with the cumin seeds, cinnamon sticks, cardamom seeds, bay leaves, and cloves.

- Red chili peppers should be crushed and halved before being added to the pan. Browning the cashews in a skillet with intermittent stirring should take about a minute. Mix thoroughly before adding to the split peas in water. If necessary, shell the peas and mash a portion of them. If necessary, taste it and season it with salt and pepper.

- Second, combine the split peas with 50 percent of the golden coconut flakes. Cover and simmer for 5 minutes. Add the remaining red pepper flakes and coconut flakes as a garnish. Just before serving, drain the liquid from the split peas cooked with bay leaves and cinnamon leaves. Split peas need to be rinsed and soaked for 15 minutes before they can be cooked in a pressure cooker. Pressure cook the drained turmeric with three cups of water.

Keep cooking for another 10 minutes to 15 minutes when the pressure indicator has reached full. Just chill down and let the pressure naturally decrease.

18. Tofu with Onion Sauce

Ingredients:

- Minced Yellow Onions
- Seeded Green Chile
- Five Garlic Cloves
- Ginger Root
- Water
- Cumin Seeds
- pod of black cardamom
- fenugreek seeds
- 1-stick of cinnamon
- vegetable oil
- red onions, finely sliced
- bell pepper
- sugar
- salt
- a quarter teaspoon of ground turmeric
- coriander, ground
- paprika or cayenne
- water
- for garnish, use lemon juice.
- 8 ounces of tempeh

Method:

- To make onion paste, combine the onion, chile, garlic, and ginger in a blender with 1/4 cup water and pulse until smooth.

- To make the sauce, mash the cumin seeds, cloves, cardamom, and fenugreek into a coarse paste. Heat a large cast-iron pot over moderate flame. Dry roast themixture for about a minute after adding the spices, or until the spices are fragrant.

- Pour the oil into the pan with the spices. Heat the oil. Add peppers, onions, sugar, and 1/4 teaspoon salt to taste. After about 20 minutes of tossing and mixing, the onions will begin to caramelize or turn golden brown. 2 teaspoons of the onion and pepper mixture can be used as a garnish.

- Combine the onion paste from Step 1 WITH the spices turmeric, coriander, paprika, and 1/2 teaspoon salt in a mixing bowl. Stir occasionally while cooking for six minutes, or until the aroma begins to waft..

- Before adding the water and steamed tempeh, give it a good stir. The heat should be adjusted to medium-low. Allow 20 minutes of cooking time for the sauce to thicken and the tempeh to absorb the sauce's color. As a garnish, place the caramelized onion on top. Serve immediately.

19. PULAO Rice Prawns Ingredients::

Ingredients:

- Shelled Prawns
- Coconut milk
- Water
- Bay leaves
- Cardamoms
- Red chili powder
- Turmeric powder
- Fresh coriander
- Garam masala
- Black pepper and pepper
- Asafetida powder
- Extra virgin olive oil

Direction:

- Put some olive oil in the frying pan. Warm it up. After that, put in the black pepper, cardamoms, bay leaves, and clove spices, and let them cook for about one to two minutes, or until the aroma is released. The tea leaf ball should also have cardamom, bay leaves, and cloves added to it. Prawns, asafoetida powder, turmeric, garam masala, chili powder, and salt should be added, and the mixture should be thoroughly combined. After draining the rice, put it in the pan and cover it with a mixture of 500 milliliters of water and 200 milliliters of coconut milk. Reduce the heat, and continue to simmer until the food is completely cooked.

- To finish, sprinkle on some fresh coriander leaves.

20. POTATO and Rosemary Risotto

Ingredients:

- Rosemary
- Chopped green onion
- Olive oil
- Arborio rice
- Yukon gold potato
- Parmesan cheese
- Chicken stock
- Butter,(Shredded)
- Pepper and salt, to taste

Direction:

- Pour some olive oil into the Dutch oven, and then heat it up over a medium-high burner. Cook the rosemary for one minute after adding it to the pan. The next step is to add the green onion and sauté it for two minutes, or until it becomes translucent.

- Decrease the flame to medium and sprinkle it with salt before serving. Allow the skin to perspire for eight minutes.

- Rice should be added once the lid is removed, the flame turned up to moderate-high, and the lid is replaced. Combine it really thoroughly. Cook for a further minute after adding the potato. After the chicken stock has been added, bring the combination to a boiling point. Turn the flame down to a gentle simmer and cook for twenty minutes, or until the pasta is firm but tender.

- Turn off the flame before adding the butter and the Parmesan. Relax for the next five minutes. If necessary, add extra of the stock. Pepper the meat with black pepper.

21. SPICY Red Lentil Cauliflower Potato Casserole

Ingredients:

- Oil
- red lentils
- chopped carrots
- salt
- ground turmeric
- powdered garlic
- garam masala
- cumin seeds
- cayenne pepper
- flakes of dried onion
- tomatoes,
- cauliflower
- salt
- fenugreek leaves
- hefty sprinkle of black pepper
- russet potatoes
- salt
- garlic powder
- coriander powder
- cayenne
- safflower oil
- chopped cilantro
- lemon juice for decoration

Method:

- Warm the oven to 400 degrees Fahrenheit. Oil the bottom of baking dish and also sides.Mix in the water, red lentils, carrot, salt, cayenne, cumin, onion flakes, turmeric, garlic, garam masala, and garam masala. Combine gently, then spread tomato slices over the lentil mixture.

- Spread the cauliflower out and then arrange the tomatoes over top. After brushing or spraying oil on the cauliflower,put some salt and pepper over it. Tear some fenugreek leaves apart using your fingers and sprinkle them over the cauliflower. Substitute 1/2 teaspoon of mustard powder for the fenugreek and sprinkle it over the cauliflower.

- Put potato pieces inside the cauliflower, using enough to cover the bottom and the sides of the dish. The potatoes will reduce in size during baking. Once you've brushed or sprayed oil on the potatoes, it's time to season them with salt, garlic powder, coriander, and cayenne.

- Water should be misted or sprinkled lightly over the potatoes. After 50 to 60 minutes in the oven, the layers of cauliflower and potatoes should be tenderenough to be pierced by a toothpick. Serve immediately while still hot, and top with fresh cilantro and lemon juice.

22. Lentil Pastries

Ingredients:

- Half a cup of red lentils
- water
- fennel seeds
- coriander seeds
- Garam Masala
- Garlic mashed
- Ginger paste
- Spicy sauce
- Vegan masala
- Garam masala
- Olive or plant oil
- Butter
- Fresh Cheese

Method:

- In a saucepan, bring the lentils and 1 cup of water to a boil to make the filling. Cook the lentils in a pan that has a lid over half of it over a medium heat until they are cooked through and the skins are just beginning to tear. After nine minutes, make sure to mix it up and check it again. If the lentils are drying out and sticking to the pan, add another tablespoon or two of water. The recommended cooking time is ten to eleven minutes. Get rid of the excess fluid, then set it to the side.
- To set up the flavor mix, heat a dish over medium intensity and dry-cook the coriander and fennel seeds for about a moment, or until the fennel seeds start to change tone. Grind the Ingredients with the cayenne, coriander, turmeric, and garam masala once they have cooled.
- Put two tablespoons of oil into a saucepan and set it over medium heat. Heat the oil in a small saucepan and add the garlic, ginger, and asafetida; sauté for one minute, or until the garlic is golden. After adding the ground flavors from Step 2, give it a good stir and let it boil for a while. Combine the cooked lentils with the salt and chat masala. After about 4 or 5 minutes, when the mixture will be brittle and some of the lentils will have

been squished, continue tossing and heating it. Salt and pepper to taste. It's best to get started on the baking while the baked products are still cool.

- The pastry dough needs to be made. It ought to become smooth if you need it for a minute. If necessary, add additional liquid to maintain a soft dough. From the dough, make spheres the size of golf balls. Roll each ball out to a diameter of four or five inches and a thickness of about one eighth of an inch on a floured surface. If you want, you can draw lopsided circles.

- Form a ball with your hands and 1.5–2 teaspoons of the lentil mixture. Spread the dough and set the filled ball on top. To secure, fold in half the length of the fabric and push down on both edges. The cake has to be pressed down gently on a baking pan lined with material. Carry on with the rest of the baked goods. The grill should be prepared to a temperature of 400 degrees Fahrenheit. Spread the oil throughout using a paintbrush or a spray bottle.

- Pastry should be baked for 20–25minutes, or until it is golden and crisp. Check the alignment of the border and the center. Right before serving, just a little. It may sit out at room temperature for a while without spoiling. Keep in the fridge for up to four days if covered. Reheat it just before serving.

23. **BUTTERNUT Coconut Red Lentil Soup**

This simple lentil soup made with butternut squash and coconut milk is perfect for fallit can be a good option for maintenance-strange

Ingredients:

- 3 medium potatoes
- One onion, skinned and divided
- Garlic mashed
- Ginger paste
- Spicy sauce
- Vegan masala
- Garam masala
- Olive or plant oil
- Butter
- Fresh Cheese
- Two tsp vinegar
- Two tbsp turmeric
- Chili powder

Method:

- First, warm the oil in a cast-iron pot over moderate flame. When the oil is warmed up, toss in the curry leaves and mustard seeds. Prepare food for thirty seconds. For about a minute, or until the garlic is golden, sauté the asafetida with the finely chopped garlic. After five-minutes, remove the lid, give everything a good stir, and then add the squash. The coconut, chili powder, and garam masala need to be mixed together so that they are evenly coated.

- Second, put the drained lentils back in the pot. When you add the salt, water, and coconut milk, be sure to mix it well. After warming up to a boiling point, cover and cook for seven minutes. Cover and cook over low flame for 13–16 minutes, or until the squash and lentils are tender. Garnish with fresh juice of lemon and chopped cilantro and serve.

24. CAULIFLOWER Dipped in Curry-sauce

Ingredients::

- head of cauliflower
- 3–4 quarts of water
- salt
- turmeric
- cayenne
- oil for the sauce
- ginger
- 6 cloves garlic
- Red pepper flakes,
- onion
- garam masala
- cumin powder
- coriander powder
- turmeric (2 1/2 cups)
- tomatoes
- Salt, to taste
- maple syrup
- dried fenugreek leaves
- 6 ounces of vegan coconut milk
- soaked cashews in water

Method:

- In a large pot, heat a lot of water. Submerge the cauliflower fully in water. Add salt, turmeric, and cayenne pepper (if using) to the water. Submerge the cauliflower in a pot of vigorously summering water. Cook for another 3 minutes under the cover after 3 minutes under the cover. Blanching ensures that the cauliflower's center is properly cooked when roasting.

- Oil should be heated over a moderate flame in a big cast-iron pot.Fry till shallots are golden. Put the ginger, garlic, chile and sauté for 2 minutes. While mixing, Indian spice blend, cumin, coriander, and turmeric powder are added. Tomatoes,salt, sugar, and fenugreek leaves are all recommended. Cover and boil for 8 to 9 minutes, stirring occasionally, until saucy. The larger bits of tomato are crushed.

- After a brief chilling period, transfer to a blender. Blend in the cashews and coconut milk until smooth and gooey. A few tablespoons of water can be added if the sauce is very thick. Set aside after tasting and adjusting the salt and spices as needed. The oven should be warmed to a temperature of 400 degrees Fahrenheit.

- If preferred, apply oil to the roasting pan.Place the blanched cauliflower in the roasting pan. Add some purée in between the florets by splitting them with your hands and allowing the sauce to sink in. Pour the thick puree slowly over the top of the cauliflower, coating the entire head. Some sauce will fall to the side. Save approximately a third or a quarter of the sauce to serve as a side dish later.

- Bake for 30 minutes, then flip the dish over, top with more sauce, and bake for another 15 minutes. Bake the cauliflower until it is dry to the touch, check if it's fully cooked with the help of a fork and the sauce on the side begins to thicken.

- Over medium temperature, bring the remaining sauce to the boiling point and serve on the side. Blanched veggies can be added to the sauce if desired. To serve, slice a large amount of cauliflower. Dress with sauce.

25. **TEMPEH in Onion Sauce**

Ingredients:

- minced yellow onions
- seeded green chili
- five garlic cloves
- ginger root
- water
- cumin seeds
- pod of black cardamom
- Fenugreek seeds
- 1-STICK of cinnamon
- Vegetable oil
- red onions, finely sliced
- bell pepper
- sugar
- salt
- A quarter teaspoon of ground turmeric

- coriander, ground
- paprika or cayenne
- water
- For garnish, use lemon juice.
- 8 ounces of tempeh

Method:

- To make onion paste, combine the onion, chili, garlic, and ginger in a blender with 1/4 cup water and pulse until smooth.
- To make the sauce, mash the cumin seeds, cloves, cardamom, and fenugreek into a coarse paste. Heat a large cast-iron pot over moderate flame. Dry roast the mixture for about a minute after adding the spices, or until the spices are fragrant.
- Pour the oil into the pan with the spices. Heat the oil. Add peppers, onions, sugar, and 1/4 teaspoon salt to taste. After about 20 minutes of tossing and mixing, the onions will begin to caramelize or turn golden brown. 2 teaspoons of the onion and pepper mixture can be used as a garnish.
- Combine the onion paste from Step 1 WITH the spices turmeric, coriander, paprika, and 1/2 teaspoon salt in a mixing bowl. Stir occasionally while cooking for six minutes, or until the aroma begins to waft..
- Before adding the water and steamed tempeh, give it a good stir. The heat should be adjusted to medium-low. Allow 20 minutes of cooking time for the sauce tothicken and the tempeh to absorb the sauce's color. As a garnish, place the caramelized onion on top. Serve immediately.

Chapter 4

Low-fiber diet

26. LOW-FIBER Omelet

You may get a good head start on the day by following this recipe for an omelet that is low in fiber. This recipe will create one dish for you (one omelet), but you are more than welcome to multiply the Ingredients in order to store some for later use.

Ingredients:

- salt
- pepper
- whole egg, four large egg whites, separated from the yolk
- unsalted butter
- shredded mozzarella cheese

Direction:

- Make a mixture of one whole egg and four egg whites by whisking them together in a medium-sized container. Incorporate the addition of ground black pepper and sodium chloride into the mix.

- After that, place a frying pan over a heat setting that is somewhere in the middle between medium and low, and then place a sufficient amount of butter into the iron-cast pot. Once the butter has undergone the process of meltdown, add the Ingredients from the medium-sized bowl, which contains the eggs, salt, and pepper, to the mixture. Proceed with the process after the butter has been melted.

- After the frying step, distribute the contents of a quarter cup of mozzarella cheese in a uniform manner across one side of the omelet. It is recommended that the omelet be folded in half, specifically over the cheese, in order to make the melting process of the cheese go more smoothly.

- Put the finished product on a plate, and then savor the experience of eating it.

27. LOW-FIBER Tofu

The vast majority of people find it repugnant to consider the possibility of swallowing cubes made of synthetic flesh. This is not something that is difficult to understand.

After all, they're just cubes made out of some kind of fake meat. In spite of this, what sets these apart from the others is the fact that they are good imitation meat cubes, which is, in the end, all that really matters. The following recipe for tofu yields a total of 4 servings, so please plan accordingly.

Ingredients:

- maple syrup
- lemon juice
- soy sauce
- Ten grams of extra-firm tofu garlic powder
- coconut oil
- sriracha

Direction:

- Get a bowl that is about the right size for you. Blend the lemon juice, soy sauce, maple syrup, and sriracha in there, along with the tofu and garlic powder.

- Gently stir in this mixture so that the shape of the tofu is not compromised in any way. The goal here is to coat the tofu cubes with the remaining Ingredients as thoroughly as possible. Allow this to sit for a while, approximately fifteen minutes, and stir it every so often while it's sitting there.

- Place a cast-iron saucepan on the gas and turn the flame to medium. Add the coconut oil to the pan. After this has melted, add the tofu cubes to the pan and allow them to cook for a total of three minutes on each side. If there is any

remaining mixture in the bowl, put it in the pot and continue to sear the tofu for an additional minute on each side.

- You may now enjoy the tofu by placing it on a platter and serving it to yourself. After you've had a few bites, you'll understand what I meant when I referred to "good meat cubes."

28. Low-fiber banana smoothie

The term "simple" may potentially be an understatement when describing the level of complexity associated with this particular dish. This recipe is characterized by its simplicity, delectable taste, and convenience of requiring only two readily available Ingredients. The combination of bananas and ice is a popular choice among individuals seeking a refreshing and nutritious treat. While some individuals may perceive bananas as having a consistent fiber content, the quantity employed in this particular recipe enables it to be categorized as low-fiber, especially containing less than around 5 grams per serving.

Ingredients:

- A whole banana, frozen
- Ice cubes

Direction:

- Once again, it might be argued that the term "simple" is an oversimplification. To prepare the smoothie, the frozen banana and ice should be placed in a blender and blended until the mixture reaches a smoothie-like consistency.
- While one may be tempted to incorporate protein powder into this beverage, it is advisable to refrain from doing so due to its potential drawbacks and limited overall benefits. In addition to its elevated protein content, protein powder generally exhibits a substantial concentration of dietary fiber. In the event of any ambiguity, it is advisable to consult the nutritional information provided on the label of the protein powder. The use of additional Ingredients is permissible, provided that the amount per serving does not exceed 2 grams.

However, exceeding the prescribed limit will result in non-compliance with the low-fiber phase.

29. Homemade Apple-sauce

The homemade applesauce that you can produce with the help of this foolproof recipe is as delectable as it is simple to prepare. Who doesn't adore a good serving of applesauce? You will end up with a total of 12 cups of it if you follow this recipe, so even if you only make it once, you will have plenty for a considerable amount of time.

Ingredients:

- One unit of measurement equivalent to a cup of apple cider or apple juice serving as a suitable substitute
- apples that have been peeled and sliced into eight pieces for each apple
- cinnamon
- brown sugar
- A lemon

Direction:

- Gather your Ingredients and place them in a pot. Nutmeg and butter are optional additions, depending on taste. Twenty-five minutes of cooking time should be allotted for this concoction over medium heat.

- After that's done, toss everything into a blender or food processor and whirl it around until it's completely smooth. The finished product can be stored in the refrigerator until it is ready to be eaten. Believe me, this apple sauce is mouth-watering.

30. Baked Salmon with Rosemary and Lemon

If you are a more experienced cook than the average person who makes macaroni and cheese, you probably crave a bit more of a challenge than what you are currently confronting in the kitchen. There's no need to look any further. After completing this baked salmon with rosemary dish, you will have a total of two servings. Please, do not wait much longer; now we may start.

Ingredients:

- Two salmon fillets with the bones and skin removed
- Rosemary taste test to find the
- lemon
- A teaspoon of olive oil
- Coarse salt

Directions:

- Prepare a temperature in the oven of 400 degrees Fahrenheit by reheating it. Take half of the lemon slices and place them across the bottom of a baking dish.

- Next, sprinkle two sprigs of rosemary over the top of the lemon slices. After that, take your salmon fillets and lay them on top of the lemon slices that you've just laid out. This will be the next step in the process. Place the tworemaining sprigs of rosemary and the remaining two slices of lemon on top of the fillets.

- The dish that you have just made ought to be able to be characterized as a "lemon and rosemary sandwich with salmon in the middle." Last but not least, pour some olive oil over the tops of these sandwiches made with lemon andsalmon.

- Reheat the oven to 400 degrees and place a microwaveable dish inside. Cook for twenty minutes. Prepare according to taste. Enjoy!

31. Lemon Chicken Breasts

The meat recipe to be discussed pertains to chicken, which is widely recognized as one of the most commonly consumed meats globally. The perception that foreign cuisines often resemble the flavour of chicken can be attributed to an individual'sextensive exposure to chicken, leading to a cognitive adjustment of their taste buds. This culinary formula for exceptional lemon-infused chicken breasts will produce a total of four individual portions.

Ingredients:

- One teaspoon of minced garlic
- a quantity of melted butter equivalent to three teaspoons.
- A quantity of chicken broth measuring one-fourth cup and a quantity of lemon juice measuring 2 teaspoons
- one teaspoon of Italian seasoning. The salt and pepper should be subjected to a tasting test in order to get a desired flavour profile that aligns with personal preferences.
- one tablespoon of olive oil.
- The recipe calls for 1 tablespoon of minced parsley and 1.5 pounds of skinless, boneless chicken breasts.

Direction:

- It is recommended to apply a seasoning mixture consisting of salt, pepper, and Italian seasoning to both sides of the chicken breasts. The oven should be reheated to a temperature of 400 degrees Fahrenheit, and a large frying pan should be obtained. Incorporate the olive oil into the mixture. After heating the olive oil to an appropriate temperature, proceed to place the chicken breasts into the pot.
- Cook each side of the chicken breasts for 4 minutes. Transfer the chicken to a baking dish that is a suitable size.
- First, acquire a bowl and proceed to amalgamate the chicken broth, garlic, lemon juice, and butter. Once the mixture has achieved a homogeneous consistency, proceed to coat the chicken breasts with it.
- The recommended duration for baking the chicken breasts is around 30 minutes, or until they have reached a fully cooked state. After the completion of the cooking process, take out the chicken from the oven and employ a

spoon to extract a portion of the sauce that has gathered at the base, thereafter redistributing it evenly onto the chicken.

- Gently distribute the parsley evenly atop the chicken breasts and savour the culinary experience.

32. Baked Spaghetti Squash with Parmesan Cheese

It is possible that meat consumption may not align with your dietary preferences or needs. While I may not possess a complete personal understanding of your perspective, I am able to offer different viewpoints or options for consideration. The following recipe outlines the preparation of baked spaghetti squash accompanied by parmesan cheese, yielding a total of six servings.

Ingredients:

- pepper
- Salt
- Parmesan cheese
- Butter
- Spaghetti
- Squash

Direction:

- Initially, it is recommended to set the temperature of the oven to 375 degrees Fahrenheit.

- To prepare the spaghetti squash, it is recommended to puncture the surface with a knife, creating a series of small holes. Ensure that the holes are evenly distributed throughout the squash. Utilize a baking dish as the receptacle for the squash and subject it to a baking process for approximately fifty minutes, or until it reaches a state of tenderness.

- After the squash has been roasted, it should be sliced into halves, and all of the seeds should be removed by scooping them out. Please obtain a bowl and a fork and proceed to extract the squash by scraping it into the bowl, ensuring that the resulting strands are lengthy and meaty in nature. The butter should be melted and incorporated into the bowl, followed by the combination of the squash and parmesan, which should also be mixed together.

- Finally, season the ultimate preparation with salt and pepper, and savour it while it is still hot.

33. Pork Chop

Pork chops are a popular meat dish that is commonly consumed in various culinary traditions around the world. During the concluding phase of the diverticulitis diet, a significant number of meats are deemed unsuitable due to their propensity to induce inflammation. It is advisable to address one's carnivorous inclination in a timelymanner. What more effective approach could be employed than utilizing pork chops?

This particular recipe for pork chops has the capacity to produce a total of four servings.

Ingredients:

- Butter,

- olive oil
- Garlic powder
- Honey
- Minced garlic
- Water
- Salt
- Pepper
- Pork chops
- White vinegar

Direction:

- Raise the temperature of your grill to medium-high. Sprinkle all of the spices, including the garlic powder, pepper, and salt, over the pork chops before cooking them. The olive oil should be heated in the skillet over a heat setting of medium to medium-high. To cook the pork chops, sear them on both sides for around 4 to 5 minutes. After that, arrange the chops in a single layer on a platter and set them aside for a short while you move on to the nextstage.

- Then, proceed to add the garlic to the same skillet after reducing the heat to medium. Sauté the Ingredients for about 30 seconds, or until the aroma of garlic can be detected. After that, pour in the water, honey, and vinegar, and

continue to whisk as the mixture continues to cook for about another four minutes.

- Put the pork chops back into the pan and coat them in a good amount of the sauce that you've just made before placing them back in the oven. The pork chops should then be grilled for one to two minutes. Pork is one of the most dangerous types of meat when it comes to parasites, so you need to make sure that the inside of your chops is grey before you consume them. Place on a platter, and bask in the satisfaction of having your carnivorous itch scratched!

34. Smoked Turkey-Wrapped Zucchini Sticks

It is possible that meat consumption may not align with your dietary preferences or needs. While I may not possess a complete personal understanding of your perspective, I am able to offer different viewpoints or options for consideration. The following recipe outlines the preparation of smoked turkey wrapped in zucchini,which can be used for a total of four servings.

Ingredients:

- Smoked turkey
- Zucchini (2)
- Packed arugula (1 cup)

- Salt

Direction:
- Place smoked turkey on your work surface.
- Top with the zucchini, arugula, and salt.
- Wrap your turkey around vegetables.
- Repeat with your remaining Ingredients
- Serve it.
- Enjoy!

35. Balsamic Chicken, Tomatoes, and White Bean Salad

The meat recipe to be discussed pertains to chicken, which is widely recognized as one of the most commonly consumed meats globally. The perception that foreign cuisines often resemble the flavor of chicken can be attributed to an individual'sextensive exposure to chicken, leading to a cognitive adjustment of their taste buds. This culinary formula for exceptional balsamic chicken, tomatoes, and white bean salad will produce a total of four individual portions.

Ingredients:
- Fat mayonnaise (1/2 cup)
- Finely cleaved little onion (1 pc.)
- Finely hacked celery stems (1 pc.)
- Minced garlic (1 clove)
- Ground dark pepper (1/8 tsp.)
- Hacked parsley (1 tbsp.)
- Salt (1/8 tsp.)
- Depleted kippers or smoked herring (1 6-oz. pc.)
- Lemon juice (1 tsp.)

Direction:
- Mix together every one of the fixings aside from the kipper in a medium-sized bowl.
- Add chipped kippers to the blend and tenderly throw them.
- Refrigerate once the plate of mixed greens is finished. You can use it as a sandwich filling or as a side dish to your primary course.

36. CHICKEN Cacciatore

Ingredients:

- Finely hacked celery stem (1 pc.)
- Lemon juice (one teaspoon.)
- Minced garlic (1 clove)
- Plain breadcrumbs (1 cup)
- Whole wheat burger buns
- Vegetable stock (5 cups)
- Squeezed orange (2 cups)
- Hacked parsley (one tablespoon)

Direction:

- Preheat the broiler to 400°F. Strip and cut yams into tiny pieces.
- Arrange the yams on a sheet of baking parchment and coat them evenly with salt, pepper and olive oil.
- Cook the potatoes in the broiler for 45–50 minutes at 400°F, or until the yams are very caramelized. Put away.
- In an enormous soup pot, cook the leeks or onions over moderate to high heat for 8 minutes or until they are delicate.
- Add the white wine and heat it to the point of boiling until the wine vanishes.
- Whenever all the wine has dissipated, add the vegetable stock, thyme, and yams, and then, at that point, bring the entire soup blend into a bubble.
- Turn down the heat and let it stew for 20 minutes, or until the vegetables are delicate.
- Utilise a blender to puree the soup in clusters. Warm each group of soups prior to serving.

37. CHICKEN Adobo

Ingredients:

- Hacked little onion (1 pc.)
- Chopped jalapeno (1 pc.)
- Mashed cumin (2 tsp.)
- Diced garlic (2 tsp.)
- Crushed dark beans (2 14.5 oz. jars)
- Raw yam (2 cups)

- Beaten egg (1 pc.)
- Plain breadcrumbs (1 cup)
- Whole wheat burger buns
- Deli-cooked roasted turkey (1 WHOLE)
- Whole wheat, or a combination of grains (6 pcs.)

Direction:
- Mix together every one of the fixings aside from the kipper in a medium-sized bowl.
- Add chipped kippers to the blend and tenderly throw them.
- Refrigerate once the plate of mixed greens is finished. You can use it as a sandwich filling or as a side dish to your primary course.

38. Chicken and Bell Pepper Sauté

Ingredients:
- Hacked little onion (1 pc.)
- Chopped jalapeno (1 pc.)
- Mashed cumin (2 tsp.)
- Finely hacked celery stem (1 pc.)
- Hacked parsley (1 tbsp.)
- Finely chopped garlic (one clove)
- Deli-cooked roasted turkey (1 WHOLE)
- Whole wheat or a combination of grains (6 pcs.)
- Lemon juice (one tsp.)

Direction:
- Preheat the grill.
- Combine the egg whites, cereal, and onions. Furthermore, ¼ cup fruit purée. Add the chicken. Blend everything well and make a burger patty.
- Shower non-stick covering on the oven skillet. Put the burger on the rack and cook for around 5 minutes prior to turning over. Sear for an additional 5 minutes, or, on the other hand, until the meat is, at this point, not pinkish in shading.
- Heat the remainder of the fruit purée and pour it over the burger.
- While the burger is still cooking, whisk together some dressing fixings for certain pounded strawberries.

- Get a plate of mixed greens in a bowl and blend the tomato, onion, and strawberries together. Shower with a dressing. Serve.

39. CHICKEN Stir-fry

Ingredients:
- Hacked little onion (1 pc.)
- Chopped jalapeno (1 pc.)
- Mashed cumin (2 tsp.)
- Finely hacked celery stem (1 pc.)
- Lemon juice (two tsp.)
- Minced garlic (one clove)
- Deli-cooked roasted turkey (1 WHOLE)
- Whole wheat or a combination of grains (6 pcs.)
- Plain breadcrumbs (1 cup)
- Hacked parsley (one tbsp.)

Direction:
- Shower non-stick covering on the oven skillet. Put the burger on the rack and cook for around 5 minutes prior to turning over.
- Sear for an additional 5 minutes, or, on the other hand, until the meat is, at this point, not pinkish in shading.
- Put the combination in the cooler to save.
- In the interim, add salt, vinegar, cabbage, and cayenne pepper to a different blending bowl. Throw the cabbage in to blend it in with different fixings.
- Discard both the skin and osseous components of the broiled poultry, and proceed with cutting the chicken into smaller pieces.
- Add the chicken to the mayonnaise blend and join it.
- Orchestrate the cabbage and the chicken equitably in the flatbread cuts and roll them firmly.
- You can either eat it all alone or heat it using a toaster or microwave.

40. ROSEMARY Chicken

Ingredients:

- Soft chicken breast, 112 pounds
- Olive oil for cooking, (two tablespoons)
- Leaves of rosemary , (finely cut)
- Sea-salt
- Pickles liquid
- Black pepper
- Red cabbage, chopped
- Freshly ground pepper

Direction:

- The oven has preheated to 420 degrees Fahrenheit.
- Place the chicken chunks on a baking tray with a rim.
- Spray with olive oil and season with oregano, salt, and chilli.
- Cook for 15–20 minutes, or until liquids flow clean.

41. Turkey and Kale Sauté

Ingredients:

- Hacked little onion (1 pc.)
- Chopped jalapeno (1 pc.)
- Bell pepper
- Black pepper
- Red cabbage, chopped
- Turkey (1 WHOLE)
- Kale
- Green beans
- Oil
- Stir-fry sauce

Direction:

- Because of how quickly stir-fries move, all of the chopping and mincing should be done before beginning the cooking process. Green beans should have their ends trimmed and chopped off; bell peppers should be sliced; kale should becut into halves; and garlic and ginger should be minced. If you are not using a kale and cabbage mixture that has already been prepared, you will need to chop the necessary quantities of each individual item.

- Mix the hoisin sauce, agave nectar (or honey), water, and soy sauce together in a bowl using a whisk. Put it to the side until you are ready to add it to thestir-fry, and then set it aside.

- Bring a large pot that does not stick to the pan to medium-high heat. Add the ground turkey to the pan after giving it a light coating of cooking spray. While the turkey is cooking, use a spatula made of wood or silicone to break it upinto smaller pieces. When the turkey is done cooking all the way through, remove it from the oven and place it in a bowl using a slotted spoon.

- Garlic and ginger are being stir-fried with green beans and red bell peppers in a skillet made of nonstick material.

- In order to cook the vegetables, first put the avocado oil and the sesame oil in the pot. After adding the green beans to the pan, continue to cook for another two minutes while swirling the pan occasionally. Cook the red bell pepper and kale for one minute after adding them to the pan. Last but not least, stir in the ginger and garlic, and continue to heat for up to a minute while being careful not to let the garlic burn.

- It's time to put everything together, so let's combine our efforts! Place the ground turkey back into the skillet and add the kale and cabbage mixture along with the sauce at the same time. Cook everything for approximately a minute, until it is completely warmed through and the kale or cabbage has become somewhat wilted.

- SERVE over a bed of rice, quinoa, or cauliflower rice and top with the stir-fried turkey.

42. **Turkey with Bell Peppers and Rosemary**

Ingredients:

- Chopped jalapeno (1 pc.)
- Pickles liquid
- Black pepper
- Red cabbage, chopped
- Whole wheat burger buns
- Deli-cooked roasted turkey (1 WHOLE)
- Vegetable stock (5 cups)
- Squeezed orange (2 cups)

Direction:

- Preheat the broiler to 400°F. Strip and cut yams into tiny pieces.
- Put the yams on a baking parchment and session them with pepper, olive oil and salt.

- Cook the potatoes in the broiler for 45–50 minutes at 400°F, or until the yams are very caramelized. Put away.
- In an enormous soup pot, cook the leeks or onions over moderate to high flame for 8 minutes or until they are delicate. Put garlic and ginger and mix and cook for another moment. Pour the white wine and heat it to the point of boiling until the wine vanishes.
- Whenever all the wine has dissipated, add the vegetable stock, thyme, and yams, and then, at that point, bring the entire soup blend into a bubble.
- Turn down the heat and let it stew for 20 minutes, or until the vegetables are delicate.
- Utilise a blender to puree the soup in clusters. Warm each group of soups prior to serving.

43. Easy Ground Turkey and Spinach Stir-Fry

Ingredients:
- Hacked little onion (1 pc.)
- Spinach
- Chopped jalapeno (1 pc.)
- Bell pepper
- Black pepper
- Red cabbage, chopped
- Turkey (1 WHOLE)
- Oil
- Stir-fry sauce

Direction:
- Because of how quickly stir-fries move, all of the chopping and mincing should be done before beginning the cooking process. Green beans should have their ends trimmed and chopped off; bell peppers should be sliced; spinach should be blanched and cut; and garlic and ginger should be minced. If you are notusing a kale and cabbage mixture that has already been prepared, you will need to chop the necessary quantities of each individual item.
- Mix the hoisin sauce, agave nectar (or honey), water, and soy sauce together in a bowl using a whisk. Put it to the side until you are ready to add it to thestir-fry, and then set it aside.
- Bring a large pot that does not stick to the pan to medium-high heat. Add the ground turkey to the pan after giving it a light coating of cooking spray. While the turkey is cooking, use a spatula made of wood or silicone to break it upinto smaller pieces. When the turkey is done cooking all the way through, remove it from the oven and place it in a bowl using a slotted spoon.

- Garlic and ginger are being stir-fried with green beans and red bell peppers in a skillet made of nonstick material.
- In order to cook the vegetables, first put the avocado oil and the sesame oil in the skillet. After adding the green beans to the pan, continue to cook for another two minutes while swirling the pan occasionally. Cook the red bell pepper and spinach for one minute after adding them to the pan. Last but not least, stir in the ginger and garlic, and continue to heat for up to a minutewhile being careful not to let the garlic burn.
- It's time to put everything together, so let's combine our efforts! Place the ground turkey back into the skillet and add the kale and cabbage mixture along with the sauce at the same time. Cook everything for approximately a minute, until it is completely warmed through and the kale or cabbage has become somewhat wilted.
- SERVE over a bed of rice, quinoa, or cauliflower rice and top with the stir-fried turkey.

44. Rosemary Chicken Stew

Ingredients:

- Soft chicken breast, 112 pounds
- Two tablespoons of sea salt
- A teaspoons of freshly powered black peppercorns
- Olive oil, two tablespoons
- 2 tablespoons fresh rosemary leaves, chopped

Direction:

- The oven has preheated to 425 degrees Fahrenheit.
- Place the chicken chunks on a baking tray with a rim.
- Spray some olive oil and add the herbs and spices like oregano, salt, and chilli.
- Cook for twenty minutes, or until liquids flow clean.

45. Same Miso Chicken

Ingredients:

- Hacked little onion (1 pc.)
- Chopped jalapeno (1 pc.)
- Mashed cumin (2 tsp.)
- Chopped jalapeno (1 pc.)
- Pickles liquid
- Black pepper
- Red cabbage, chopped

- Whole wheat burger buns
- Deli-cooked roasted turkey (1 WHOLE)

Direction:

- In a specious nonstick pot over moderately-high flame, warm the olive oil until it shimmers.
- Marinate the chicken with salt,black peppercorns etc.
- Place the item onto the cast-iron pot and proceed to cook for approximately four minutes on each side until the juices are transparent.
- While the chicken cooks, in a food processor/blender, combine the mayonnaise and 2 red pepper pieces.
- Blend until smooth. Place the sauce evenly onto the surface of the buns and top with the remaining roasted red pepper slices.
- Place the chicken on top.

46. Chicken Slow Cooker

Ingredients:

- Twelve large bone-in chicken thighs
- Olive oil
- Spanish onion
- Chorizo picante
- Peppers,
- chicken stock
- Spanish pimento pepper filled with green olives
- tomato purée
- White wine (serve the rest of the bottle with the meal)

Direction:

- Begin by heating two tablespoons of olive oil in a generously sized pot. Sauté one Spanish onion, sliced, for approximately five minutes or until it reaches a golden hue.
- The second step,pour the contents into the pot for slow-cooking;use a 7-litre model.Begin by sautéing a total of twelve boneless chicken thighs with skin

intact, along with 225G of chorizo picante that has been thickly sliced. Cook these Ingredients in the same cast-iron pot until they exhibit a visually appealing coloration. It is important to note that this process will need to be executed in two separate batches.

- Place into the slow cooker 3 peppers of varying colors, which have been sliced into chunks, together with 150G of Spanish pimento-packed green olives that have had their pits removed.

- Pour 300 milliliters of dry white wine, 300 milliliters of chicken stock, and one tablespoon of puréed tomato into the pan.
- Retrieve any remnants adhered to the flat surface, then transfer them into the slow cooker. Proceed to cover the slow cooker and initiate a cooking process on the low setting for a duration of six hours.

47. Chicken Thighs with Steamed Cauliflower

Ingredients:

- Tender chicken breast, 112 pounds
- 2 tablespoons fresh rosemary leaves, chopped
- 12 tablespoons of sea salt
- 18 teaspoons of freshly ground black pepper
- Two tablespoons of olive oil for cooking

Direction:

- The oven had been warmed to the temperature of 425 degrees Fahrenheit.
- Place the chicken pieces in a singular arrangement on a baking parchment paper that possesses a rim.
- Add some salt, oregano and pepper, then spray with olive oil and season with the mixture.
- Cook for fifteen to twenty minutes, or until liquids can be poured off cleanly.

48. Steamed Salmon with Lemon-Scented Zucchini

Ingredients:

- Onion (1 pc.)
- Lemon (1 pc.)
- Zucchini (2.)
- White wine (1 cup)
- Liquid (2 cups)
- Salmon Sliced Fillets (4 6-Ounce Laptops)
- Genuine Ground Salt (1/4 Tsp.)
- Mashed pepper (1/4 Tsp.)

Direction:

- Place the lemon, zucchini, onion, water, and wine in a large Dutch broiler and heat to 350°F.
- Stove's base
- Sprinkle salt and pepper over the salmon fillets. Meanwhile, cover the vegetables on the stove with a liner rack and set them aside. Place it in medium to high heat until the fluid begins to bubble.
- Decrease the heat from medium to low and cautiously place the fillets in the rack. Cover the fillets and steam them for 8–10 minutes, or until they arecooked through.
- Serve the fillets on top of the vegetables. Add poaching fluid and top it with cut olives and embellishment, whenever wanted.

49. Tomato Basil Omelet:

It's a tomato-based omelet dish that can be considered a breakfast item for the low-fiber stage.

Nutritional values:

- 21 g of protein
- 21 g fat
- 16.5 g of carbohydrates
- Calorie count:337.5 Ingredients:
- Eggs
- Basil leaves
- Pine nuts
- Whole milk
- Salt and pepper
- Olive oil
- Tomatoes

Direction:

- Eggs, milk, salt, and pepper should be whisked together in a bowl.
- Heat some oil in a cast iron of suitable size over moderate heat.
- Spread the oil by circling the cast iron. Pour the egg mixture into a cast-iron pot and turn it to evenly distribute the mixture.
- Cover half of the omelet with the tomatoes and basil. Add pepper and salt to taste. The omelet can be loosened when the eggs are done by running aspatula under it.
- Bring the unfilled side of the omelet over the top of the filling.

- Use mild pressure. Place the omelet, along with the pine nuts and basil, on a serving plate and slide it onto the table.
- Feel free to swap out the tomatoes for another vegetable. Pine nuts can beswapped out for another type of nut if desired. The nutritional value will shift, of course.

50. Eggs with greens Nutritional values:

- Calorie count: 298
- 20 g Fat
- 8g Carbohydrate
- 18 g of protein

Ingredients:

- Cooking oil
- Garlic
- Fennel
- Egg
- Lemon
- coriander seeds
- leek
- Chilli flakes
- Greek yoghourt
- spinach
- Salt

Directions:

- Heat a cast iron over a moderate flame with half of the oil.
- Put the leeks and a bit of salt to the hot oil, and simmer until the leeks are soft. Combine the fennel seeds, coriander seeds, and garlic in abowl and stir.
- Leave it in the pan for a few seconds until it starts to smell good. Toss the spinach and chilli flakes together. Turn down the heat and let the spinach wilt.
- Shift the spinach mixture to a separate side of the pan. Put the rest of the oil in the pan's centre. When the oil is ready, crack an egg directly over the pan and fry it to your liking.
- Disengage the heater.
- Whisk the yoghurt into the spinach mixture. Place the greens on a platter for serving. Taste and adjust salt and pepper. Nine, top your salad with an egg. Season the egg with salt, pepper, and chilli flakes. Toss in some lemon juice, and you're good to go.

51. White Bean Turkey Chili

Nutritional values:
- Calorie count: 364

Ingredients:
- extra-virgin olive oil
- garlic
- lean ground turkey
- cannellini beans or white kidney beans, tomato paste
- chicken base reduced-sodium
- black pepper
- garlic powder
- chilli powder
- red pepper flakes
- oregano
- onion
- orange bell pepper
- jalapeño pepper
- Canned tomatoes
- sweet corn
- water
- Salt

Process:

- Heat some oil in a large cast-iron pot over a moderate flame. Put the onion, capsicums and garlic in the pan once the oil is hot and simmer until tender. Do it frequently. Add turkey meat to the pan.

- Break up the meat into smaller pieces while you whisk. Always check that meat is done cooking before serving.

- Combine the chicken foundation, water, corn, beans, jalapenos, tomatoes,

salt, and spices. After 7 or 8 minutes of simmering with the cover on, reduce heat to low. Take off the lid and give the **Ingredients:** a thorough blending. Lower the heat to a simmer and keep an eye on it to make sure it doesn't burn; this

should take around 10 minutes.

- Heat it up.

52. Orzo Chicken Salad with Avocado Lime Dressing

Ingredients:
- small avocado
- grated lime zest
- Garlic
- Salt
- water
- lemon juice
- red pepper flakes
- whole-wheat orzo pasta
- chicken breast
- fresh cilantro
- low-fat feta cheese
- grape tomatoes
- corn kernels

Process:

- To prepare the dressing, combine the avocado, lime juice, lime zest, garlic, water, red pepper flakes, and salt in a blender. Blend until smooth. Put some in a bowl. For a couple of hours, chill undercover in the refrigerator.

- In order to make a salad, cook the orzo as directed on the package. Before draining the water, add the corn.

- Drain, then run a cold water rinse. Drain thoroughly, then add it to a bowl.

- Stir in the tomatoes, chicken, and cilantro. Put some feta on top. Spend a couple of hours relaxing.

- Add the dressing. Stir thoroughly, then plate.

53. CHICKEN Parmesan

Ingredients:

- chicken breast half
- dried breadcrumbs
- extra-virgin olive oil
- cloves of garlic
- Italian seasoning
- part-skim shredded mozzarella cheese
- pepper
- freshly grated parmesan cheese onion, chopped
- Canned tomatoes
- Fresh herbs
- Salt

Direction:

- Place the chicken in between two layers of plastic wrap and proceed to tenderize it until it reaches an approximate thickness of 14 inches.
- Incorporate pepper into the chicken.
- The parmesan, breadcrumbs, and 1 teaspoon of oil should be combined in a small container.
- Switch the oven to the broil setting and heat it to moderately high.
- Place the oven-safe cast iron with the remaining oil over a moderately high flame. After the oil has reached a suitable temperature, proceed to introduce the chicken into the cooking vessel and continue the cooking process until the underside of the chicken attains a desirable golden brown hue. Cook the chicken until golden brown on the opposite side. When you take the chicken out of the pan, set it on a dish.
- Combine the onion and garlic in the identical cooking vessel and proceed to sauté for a brief duration until they get a softened consistency.
- Stir in the tomatoes with pepper, salt, and Italian seasoning. Cook for a couple of minutes, stirring frequently.
- Include the chicken and any cooked juices in the pan. Mix thoroughly. Make sure the chicken is completely covered in sauce by turning it around in it. The heat should be turned off when it's done.

- On top of the chicken, sprinkle mozzarella cheese. Sprinkle breadcrumbs on top of the cheese. Put the ironcast in the oven and turn on the broiler for a few seconds. Take care to prevent burning.
- Add fresh herbs as a garnish before serving.

54. Buffalo Chicken

Nutritional values:

- Calorie COUNT:320

Ingredients::

- Chicken Thai or chicken breast
- Butter or oil
- Garlic powder
- Hot pepper sauce
- Coconut aminos
- Cayenne pepper
- Ranch dressing
- Sweet potato

Process:

- The best cooking appliances for this recipe are a slow cooker and a crock pot. Definitely make advantage of one if you're in possession of one. Without using a slow cooker or an instant pot, I will explain how to prepare it on the hob.
- Cayenne pepper, ghee, coconut aminos, spicy sauce, and garlic powder should be combined in a small iron skillet. The pot should be set over a low flame. Warm the ghee by stirring it.
- Heat a pan that doesn't stick over a moderate flame. Cook the chicken in a pan until the underside is golden brown, or until it reaches the desired doneness. The chicken should be flipped over and the pan covered. After the first side is browned, turn the chicken over and continue cooking until done.
- Transfer the poultry from the cast-iron and place it onto a designated surface for slicing. It is recommended to let the chicken rest for a duration of 5 minutes before initiating the slicing process. Put the chicken in the sauce. Toss together and serve over sweet potatoes and ranch dressing, if desired. There is no consideration given to the nutritional worth of ranch dressing.

55. Savory Waffles

Ingredients:
- Carrots
- Onion
- Cheese
- Eggs
- Whole-meal flour
- Sweet potato
- Salt
- Paper
- Fresh parsley

Process:
- In a bowl, mix together the carrot, cheese, sweet potato, spring onion, salt, pepper, and parsley. Set it aside for about 8 minutes to rest.
- A whole meal of flour should be added and mixed in a second. Blend in the beaten egg. Follow the manufacturer's directions to assemble and preheat your waffle maker. Four waffles can be made in a mini or regular size.
- Prepare the waffle maker by spraying it with cooking spray. Take a quarter of the mixture and put it into the waffle machine. Thin the batter if necessary to make it pourable.
- Cook the waffle for five minutes with the cover closed, or until done as desired. Set the waffle on a cooling rack after removing it from the oven. Eight, repeat the process with the remaining waffle batter. Serve.

56. Mexican Morning Eggs

Ingredients:
- Eggs (4)
- Brown rice (1 cup)
- Black beans (¾ cup)
- Cumin
- Paprika
- Chilli powder
- Salt
- Avocado

Direction:

- Combine beans, rice, and seasonings in your skillet.
- Cook over medium heat.
- In another skillet, prepare eggs.
- Add avocado over the top.
- Serve it.
- Enjoy!

Chapter 5

Full Liquid Stage

57. Banana Almond Milk Smoothie

This smoothie is an ideal option for the full liquid stage since it has a low fat level and a high fiber content, both of which contribute to a reduction in inflammation. Because of these two factors, this smoothie is an excellent choice for the full liquid stage. Two people can be fed from this recipe if it is followed precisely..

Ingredients:

- Frozen bananas
- Almond milk
- Flax seeds
- Vanilla extract
- Cinnamon

Direction :

- Put all of the Ingredients into the blender. Add a little bit of water if the mixture is too thick.
- Start the blender and run it until the mixture reaches a silky smooth consistency.
- Stop the blender to scrape down the sides as needed.
- While you are serving others, don't forget to take some time for yourself to relax and enjoy the experience.

58. Raspberry Green Tea Smoothie

This smoothie is a fantastic option for the complete liquid stage due to the fact that it contains a relatively low amount of fat and a significant amount of fiber. Both of thesefactors help to bring about a reduction in inflammation. Two people can be fed from this recipe if it is followed precisely.. After you have acquired all of the necessary components, the preparation of this recipe for a speedy and simple smoothie will take you no more than five minutes.

Ingredients:

- Green tea (12 cups)
- Frozen raspberries (2 cups)
- Banana
- Honey (1 tbsp.)
- Sugar
- Protein powder (1/4 cup) Direction
- Put all of the Ingredients into the blender at once.
- Blend the Ingredients in a blender or food processor until the sauce is very smooth and creamy.
- The purée should be poured into the glass.
- Carry it out.
- Have fun!

59. Spinach and Berries Smoothie

Two people can be fed from this recipe if it is followed precisely..

Ingredients:

- Plant-based yogurt (half cup)
- Strawberries
- Blueberries (half cup)
- Banana
- Soy milk (1/2 cup)
- Flax seeds
- Honey
- Spinach leaves (1 cup)

Direction:
- Put all of the Ingredients into the blender. Add a little bit of water if the mixture is too thick.
- Start the blender and run it until the mixture reaches a silky smooth consistency.
- Stop the blender to scrape down the sides as needed.
- Serve it chilled, and enjoy!

60. Cantaloupe Smoothie

Two people can be fed from this recipe if it is followed precisely..

Ingredients:
- Cantaloupe purée (2 cups)
- Coconut milk (1 cup)
- Tahini (1 cup)
- Maple syrup (1/4 cup)
- Cinnamon

Direction:
- Put the cantaloupe cubes in a blender.
- Add the tahini, coconut milk, maple syrup, and cinnamon.
- Blend them until smooth.
- Pour into the glasses.
- Serve it.
- Enjoy!

61. Tropical smoothie

This smoothie is full of vitamins and minerals and is also good for digestive health.

Ingredients:
- Spinach
- Water
- Pineapple
- Mango (1 cup)
- Hemp seeds (1/4 cup)
- Fresh ginger

Direction:
- In a blender, mix the pineapple, spinach, hemp seeds, water, mango, and ginger.
- Blend them until smooth.
- Pour into the two glasses.
- Serve it.
- Enjoy!

62. Blueberry smoothie

This smoothie is delicious and good for digestive health. So it is a good option.

Ingredients:
- Soy protein powder (2 tbsp)
- Frozen blueberries (1 cup)
- Soy milk (2 cups)

Direction:
- Place all Ingredients into a blender.
- Blend them properly until it's smooth.
- Serve it.
- Enjoy!

63. Greens Smoothie

Ingredients:
- Water
- Spinach leaves (1 cup)
- Kale leaves (2)
- Romaine lettuce leaves (2)
- Avocado
- Pear

Direction:
- Combine the romaine lettuce, water, avocado, spinach, kale, and pear in your blender.
- Blend them until smooth.
- Serve it.
- Enjoy!

64. Mixed Berry Smoothie

Ingredients::
- Water
- Frozen raspberries (12 cups)
- Frozen strawberries (12 cups)
- Frozen blackberries (12 cups)
- Almond butter

Direction:
- In your blender, combine all the components.
- Blend them properly.
- Serve it.
- Enjoy!

65. Strawberry-Turmeric Smoothie

This delicious drink promotes good health. So it can be a healthy, full-liquid option. This recipe can be used for three servings.

Ingredients::
- Frozen strawberries (212 cups)
- Spinach
- Milk (2 cups)
- Ground cinnamon
- Ground turmeric

Direction:
- In your blender, combine all the components.
- Blend them properly.
- Pour into the glasses.
- Serve it.
- Enjoy!

66. Blueberry Chia Seed Smoothie

This recipe can be used for four servings.

Ingredients:

- Blueberries
- Banana
- Cantaloupe
- Milk
- Greek yogurt
- Chia seeds
- Honey

Direction:

- Make a smoothie by blending together frozen blueberries, cantaloupe, Greek yogurt, and a banana. Simply add more milk or water to make the smoothie thinner to your liking.
- Blend in the chia seeds and honey, if using.
- A glass of smoothie is poured out. Put the blender full of smoothies in the fridge for 20 minutes. The chia seeds will grow in size.
- Serve.

67. Chocolate Cherry Shake

This delicious recipe can be used for four servings.

Ingredients:

- Cocoa powder (1 tbsp)
- Frozen cherries (12 cups)
- Coconut milk (1 cup)
- Vanilla extract
- Ice cubes

Direction:

- Mix all the components in your blender.
- Blend properly.
- Pour into a glass.
- Serve it.
- Enjoy!

68. Orange Apple Breakfast Shake

This recipe can be used for four servings.

Ingredients:

- Orange sections (1/2 cup)
- Almonds (2 tbsp.)
- Apple slices (half cup)
- Milk (one cup)
- Protein Powder (14G)

Direction:

- Place all the components together in your blender.
- Mix them properly.
- Pour this mixture into a glass.
- Serve it.
- Enjoy!

69. Green Tea and Ginger Shake

This recipe can be used for four servings.

Ingredients:

- Grated ginger (2 tbsp)
- Honey (2 tbsp)
- Matcha powder (2 tbsp)
- Ice cream
- Milk

Direction:

- Combine the honey, ginger, matcha, ice cream, and milk in your blender.
- Blend them until smooth.
- Serve it.
- Enjoy!

70. HOMEMADE Eggnog

This recipe is really delicious and can be used to serve four servings. **Ingredients::**

- Eggs
- Rice milk (1 cup)
- Vanilla extract
- Dash cinnamon
- Dash nutmeg
- Rum-flavored extract
- Allspice
- Ginger

Direction:

- In a blender, combine one and a half cups of milk, the sugar, the extract flavored with rum, the pudding mix, allspice, nutmeg, and ginger.
- Blend until smooth. Combine until there are no lumps.
- After the liquid has been treated until it has a smooth consistency, pour it into a pitcher (or any other container you like).
- Pour the remaining three cups of milk into the container, and then set the

container in the refrigerator so that the eggnog can sit there until it has acquired a consistency that is comparable to that of the greatest eggnog brands.

- This is the final step, but it is certainly not the least important step. Your time

spent on this should come to about an hour total. Before you serve the dish, you must always make sure that all of the components are thoroughly combined.

71. Homemade Vanilla Pudding

This recipe can be used for four servings.

Ingredients:

- Kosher salt
- cornstarch
- egg yolks
- vanilla extract
- sugar
- whole milk

Direction:

- Make sure the milk is contained in a large saucepan, and then set the temperature to medium. Put the remaining milk, cornstarch, a half teaspoon of salt, and sugar into a large bowl. Stir in the remaining milk.

- Mix all of the **Ingredients:** together with a whisk until they are completely combined. After that, pour in the egg yolks while continuing to stir the mixture in the basin.

- When the milk starts to steam, pour half of it into the bowl with the eggs and continue cooking until the eggs are done. After whisking until the mixture has a smooth consistency, transfer the contents of the bowl to the saucepan while continuing to whisk.

- Continue to cook them over medium heat while whisking them continually until they begin to boil. You should now know that you are very close to finishing; continue whisking the mixture until it has a consistency that is comparable to pudding. As soon as this is accomplished, take the pan from the heat, add the vanilla essence, and give it a thorough swirl before returning it to the flame.

- Allow the pudding to chill in the refrigerator for approximately four hours after covering the top of the container with some plastic wrap.

- The finished product ought to have a cold and thick consistency, much like one would expect from pudding.

- Before serving, make sure to give everything a good stir. Have fun!

72. COCONUT pudding

Every time I make this dish, it comes out tasting amazing. Since it does not contain any dairy, it is a wonderful option during the entirety of the liquid phase that is associated with diverticulitis. This dish can very easily be multiplied in order to serve a greater number of people at the table.

Ingredients:

- Coconut milk
- Powdered sugar
- Cornstarch
- Vanilla
- Coconut flakes
- Mango

Direction:

- Combine all of the components and place them in a deep, wide-bottomed pot.
- In order to dissolve lumps, warm coconut milk, sugar, cornstarch, and vanilla extract.
- Keep cooking it until it reaches the desired consistency.

- If you want the pudding to have a creamy texture when you serve it, either combine it or chill it for an hour before serving.
- Mango, mint, and toasted coconut should be used to garnish the cups.

73. Mango Pudding:

This recipe provides delicious results. It is a wonderful alternative for the completeliquid stage, and it does not contain any dairy products. This recipe makes enough for four individual portions.

Ingredients:
- Mango ripe
- vegan milk
- Powdered sugar
- Cornstarch
- vanilla

Direction:
- Mix all the Ingredients together and put them in a large pot.
- Warm mango pulp, vegan milk, sugar, cornstarch, and vanilla to dissolve lumps.
- Cook until the pudding thickens.
- Chill mango pudding for 1 hour or blend before serving for a creamy texture.
- Decorate cups with mango and mint.

74. ORANGE Pudding

At this point in the process, when all of the liquid has been utilized, this is an excellent choice for what to do next. This recipe produces an amount of Ingredients that issufficient for four individual servings.

Ingredients::
- Orange juice
- Gelatin or agar-agar powder
- Sugar

Direction:
- Combine all the Ingredients in a wide pot.
- Cook until the mixture thickens.
- Pour it into your favorite mold and refrigerate for two to three hours.
- Serve it chilled and enjoy.

75. Homemade Pistachio Ice-cream

This is a delicious option for the full liquid stage. This recipe can be used for four servings.

Ingredients:

- Raw pistachios,
- Raw cashews or almonds
- Coconut or almond milk
- Arrowroot or cornstarch
- Cardamom powder
- Saffron,
- Brown sugar

Direction:

- Use a grinder or blender to process the almonds and pistachios into a coarse meal.
- Place the nut meal, non-dairy milk, cornstarch, cardamom, saffron, and sugar in a blender and process until smooth. The mixture should now be added to a skillet set over medium heat. Stirring regularly to prevent burning, bring to a boil for 5 to 6 minutes. Get rid of the heat. Taste it carefully, and if necessary, adjust the sugar. Set apart for cooling.
- Pour the mixture into ice-cream molds or a bigger container after it has chilled. For a few hours, freeze. Serve after removing the mold.

76. Coconut milk ice-cream

This is a delicious option for the full liquid stage. This recipe can be used for four servings.

Ingredients:

- Coconut flesh
- Raw pistachios,
- Raw cashews or almonds
- Coconut milk
- Arrowroot or cornstarch
- Cardamom powder
- Saffron,
- Brown sugar

Method:

- Use a grinder or blender to process the coconut flesh, almonds, and pistachios into a coarse meal.

- Place the nut meal, coconut milk, cornstarch, cardamom, saffron, and sugar in a blender and process until smooth. The mixture should now be added to a skillet set over medium heat. Stirring regularly to prevent burning, bring to a boil for 5 to 6 minutes. Get rid of the heat. Taste it carefully, and if necessary, adjust thesugar. Set apart for cooling.

- Pour the mixture into popsicle molds or a bigger container after it has chilled. For a few hours, freeze. Serve after removing the mold.

77. Banana Avocado Ice-cream

This recipe provides sufficient Ingredients for four separate servings.

Ingredients:

- Banana
- Avocado
- Coconut milk or almond milk
- Brown sugar

Process:

- Use a grinder or blender to process the bananas, avocados, and milk into a coarse meal.

- Pour the mixture into a bigger container after it has chilled. For a few hours, freeze. Serve it with banana toppings.

78. Strawberry milk ice-cream

This is a delicious option for the full liquid stage. This recipe can be used for four servings.

Ingredients:

- Strawberry
- Milk
- Vanilla extract
- Almond milk
- Whipping cream
- Brown sugar

Process:

- Use a grinder or blender to process the strawberries and milk into a coarse meal. Then add vanilla extract and whipping cream and mix them well.

- Pour the mixture into a bigger container after it has chilled. For a few hours, freeze. Serve it with banana toppings.

79. Homemade mango ice cream

This is a delicious option for the full liquid stage. This recipe can be used for four servings.

Ingredients:
- Ripe Mango
- Raw pistachios,
- raw cashews or almonds
- coconut or almond milk
- arrowroot or cornstarch
- cardamom powder
- saffron,
- raw sugar

Method:
- Use a grinder or blender to process the mango, almonds, almonds and pistachios into a coarse meal.
- Place the nut meal, non-dairy milk, cornstarch, cardamom, saffron, and sugar in a blender and process until smooth. The mixture should now be added to a skillet set over medium heat. Stirring regularly to prevent burning, bring to a boil for 5to 6 minutes. Get rid of the heat. Taste it carefully, and if necessary, adjust the sugar. Set apart for cooling.
- Pour the mixture into popsicle molds or a bigger container after it has chilled. For a few hours, freeze. Serve after removing the mold.

80. Homemade Chocolate Ice Cream

This is a delicious option for the full liquid stage. This recipe can be used for four servings.

Ingredients:
- Plant-based milk
- semi-sweet chocolate
- unsweetened cocoa powder
- heavy cream
- egg yolks
- salt
- vanilla extract

Direction:

- Get a pan ready for the sauce. After adding the cocoa powder, milk, salt, andsugar, raise the temperature to medium and continue stirring the mixture. While stirring the mixture frequently, bring the liquid to a simmer. Place the egg yolksin a separate container, and using a liquid measuring cup, remove a half cup from the liquid that is simmering. Stirring constantly as you pour, gradually add this to the egg yolks. The next step is to empty the contents of this bowl into thesaucepan.

- Keep heating the mixture without allowing it to boil until it reaches the desiredconsistency of being thick. When it has reached the desired consistency, take the pan off the heat and stir in the chocolate that has been chopped. Stirring the Ingredients together will help the chocolate melt.

- The next step is to empty the contents of the pot into a sizable basin. Put a plastic wrap cover over this bowl and place it in the refrigerator so that it may get cold.

- Take the mixture out of the refrigerator when you are ready to make the ice cream and place it in the bowl of your ice cream maker. Followthe on-screen directions to operate the machine.

- At the end of the process, you will have a delectable chocolate ice cream that will stay good for about as long as you can hold off on eating it.

81. Homemade Vanilla Ice Cream

This is delicious and dairy-free, so it is a good option for the full liquid stage. This recipe can be used for four servings.

Ingredients:

- sea salt
- vanilla extract
- Cashew cream
- Plant-based milk
- sugar
- An ice cream maker of your choice

Direction:

- Pour one cup of cream into a medium pot. Add the sugar and salt to the cashew cream once it has been poured in. Just enough heat needs to be applied to this mixture in order for the sugar to completely dissolve. After removing the pan from the heat, add the remaining milk and cream and give it a good stir beforeserving. Put this concoction in the refrigerator so that it may get nice and frosty.

- When you are ready, remove the mixture from the refrigerator and give it a good stir before placing it back in the fridge. After adding the mixture, make sure to proceed in accordance with the guidelines provided by the ice cream maker's manufacturer. The completed product will be an ice cream that is sweet and airy, and it will have a vanilla flavor.

82. PUMPKIN Soup

Because it contains a considerable level of fiber, pumpkin is an excellent choice for a holiday soup because of its high fiber content.

Ingredients:

- Chopped jalapeno (1 pc.)
- Mashed cumin (2 tsp.)
- Diced garlic (2 tsp.)
- Crushed dark beans (2 14.5 oz. jars)
- Raw yam (2 cups)
- Beaten egg (1 pc.)
- Plain breadcrumbs (1 cup)
- Whole wheat burger buns
- Turmeric (1 tsp.)
- Ground cumin (1/2 tsp.)
- Ground cayenne pepper (1/4 tsp.)
- Vegetable stock or stock (6 cups)
- Lentils (1 cup)
- Flushed and depleted garbanzo beans (2 15-OZ. jars)

Direction:

- Sauté onions in a huge pot over medium-high heat for 3–4 minutes, or until the onions are delicate.

- Add celery and carrots to the pot and continue to cook for an extra five minutes. Mix in the garlic, garam masala, turmeric, cumin, and cayenne pepper into the pot and continue to cook for 30 additional seconds.

- Add the cups of stock, lentils, garbanzo beans, and tomatoes to the pot, then, at that point, continue to mix the fixings until every one of them is joined.

- Cook the stock for an hour and a half, or until the lentils are delicate.

- For a creamier and thicker soup, you can take out a portion of the stock, puree it with a food processor, then, at that point, set it back into the pot and mix.

83. SPINACH Soup

Spinach is considered a highly favorable dietary option due to its notable fiber content, which facilitates the formation of voluminous stools and promotes their smoother passage through the digestive system. Moreover, spinach is a highly commendable provider of antioxidants, which, upon ingestion, might aid in the reduction of systemicinflammation. Moreover, spinach is a highly commendable provider of essential nutrients, including vitamins A and C, renowned for their capacity to enhance the immune system's resilience and aid in the prevention of infections.

Ingredients:

- Spinach
- water
- Onion
- vegetable broth
- black pepper
- Salt

Direction:

- Combine the spinach using a handheld immersion blender.
- Incorporate the additions of pepper and salt into the mixture, allowing it to simmer until it reaches the desired consistency.

84. TOMATO Soup

There are several mechanisms through which tomatoes can provide benefits to those suffering from diverticulitis. Tomatoes provide a notable fiber content, exhibiting potential for promoting regularity within the digestive system and mitigating thelikelihood of constipation, a prevalent catalyst for the exacerbation of diverticulitis. Tomatoes provide a valuable dietary supply of vitamins A and C, both of which play a crucial role in supporting optimal immune system functioning. In conclusion, the presence of lycopene in tomatoes has been found to possess anti-inflammatoryproperties. For safety precautions, it is advisable to extract the pips from tomatoes prior to consuming the meat. In the event that canned tomatoes are employed, it is advisable to separate the liquid from the seeds by means of straining.

Ingredients:

- Canned tomatoes crushed
- red bell pepper
- Half leek
- olive oil
- vegetable broth

- water
- dried thyme
- Salt
- pepper

Direction:
- To create a smooth mixture, employ a hand blender to combine tomatoes, leeks, and bell pepper.
- Incorporate water, broth, pepper, and salt into the mixture.
- Allow the mixture to reach the desired consistency through the process of boiling.

85. KALE Soup

Due to its anti-inflammatory properties, kale has the potential to assist in the management of symptoms associated with diverticulitis. Additionally, kale soup is devoid of fat content and boasts a significant concentration of essential elements, including iron.

Ingredients:
- Gently butter-fried yellow onion
- vegetable broth
- water
- Black pepper
- salt

Direction:
- Chop the pre-cooked kale and place it in a saucepan alongside.
- Blend using a hand blender.
- Allow the mixture to reduce until it reaches the desired consistency.

86. Beans Soup

Beans are considered a significant dietary source of fiber, which is particularlyimportant for individuals with diverticulosis. The increased fiber content of this soup can be attributed to the use of beans and brown rice.

Ingredients:
- bacon
- garlic
- shallots
- carrots

- kidney beans
- cooking brown rice
- beef broth
- bay leaves
- dried basil

Direction :

- In a sizable soup pot, proceed to cook the bacon over moderate heat until it reaches a crisp texture. Break apart and place in a separate container.
- In the identical skillet containing the rendered bacon fat, proceed to sauté the minced garlic, finely chopped shallots, and sliced carrots until they reach a state of tenderness, which typically takes approximately 5 minutes.
- Transfer the beans into a blender and process until a smooth consistency is achieved. Incorporate the veggie mixture into the pan.
- Include the bacon, rice, broth, bay leaves, and basil in the mixture. Agitate the soup mixture and elevate the temperature of the pot until it reaches a state of boiling.
- Simmer the mixture under cover, applying heat, until the rice reaches a state of

tenderness, which typically takes approximately 20 minutes. So as to accomplish a goal or complete an assignment.

87. CARROT Soup

The level of spiciness can be modified according to the type of curry, while this delicious soup exhibits an intensified essence of carrot.

Ingredients:

- olive oil
- carrots
- onion
- garlic cloves
- curry powder
- chicken broth
- carrot juice

Direction :

- Heat oil over medium heat in a large soup pot.

- Incorporate carrots and onion into the mixture and proceed with the cooking process for approximately 6 to 8 minutes. Incorporate garlic and curry powder into the mixture and continue cooking for an additional minute.

- Subsequently, incorporate broth and half a teaspoon of salt, and proceed to

simmer the mixture over a gentle heat. Place a lid on the pot and let the mixture simmer for approximately 15 minutes.

- Incorporate carrot juice into the mixture and thoroughly blend. The soup should be blended in a blender, taking into consideration the need to operate in batches. Reintroduce the soup back into the pan and proceed to season it with appropriate amounts of salt and pepper. So as to accomplish a goal or complete an assignment.

- It is worth mentioning that to enhance the texture, it is possible to incorporate a small amount of cream.

88. Mushroom and Ginger Soup

This delicious soup with an Asian influence, incorporating the flavors of garlic and ginger, has the potential to captivate individuals.

Ingredients:
- vegetable oil
- Garlic cloves
- fresh ginger
- white mushrooms
- vegetable broth
- low-sodium soy sauce
- bean sprouts
- whole wheat thin pasta
- fresh cilantro

Direction:

- Heat a substantial quantity of water with added salt until it reaches its boiling point. Incorporate pasta into the culinary preparation and proceed to cook it in accordance with the guidelines provided on the packaging, ensuring that it

reaches the desired state of firmness known as "al dente." The process of removing liquid or other substances from an area or object

- Heat oil over moderate to high temperatures in a large soup pot. Incorporate Ingredients such as garlic, ginger, and mushrooms. Continuously agitate the mixture until it reaches a state of tenderness, often requiring a duration of approximately 3 to 4 minutes.

- Incorporate vegetable stock into the mixture and raise the heat until it reaches a boiling point. Incorporate soy sauce and bean sprouts into the mixture and proceed with the cooking process until the Ingredients reach a desired level oftenderness.
- To serve, transfer the cooked noodles into separate bowls and carefully pour the soup over them. Freshly chopped cilantro is an option for garnishing the meal.

Chapter 6

Clear Liquid Stage

89. Bone Broth

Bone broth is a good option for the clear liquid stage. The reason behind choosing it as the first recipe on this list is because of its high nutritional value. This bone broth (stock) recipe makes around twelve servings.

Ingredients:

- A large onion
- water
- 2-3 pounds of bones These can be pork, chicken, or beef.
- spring onions
- ginger
- Carrot
- garlic

Directions:

- In the event that a smaller pot is used, it may be necessary to fragment the bones into smaller segments to accommodate their size. The bones need to be fully immersed in the filtered water to a minimum depth of one inch subsequent to the pouring of water into the container.
- Place the pot on the burner and regulate the heat to its maximum setting. Following a brief five-minute period of boiling, during which the undesirable substances are given an opportunity to detach from the bones and ascend to the uppermost layer, proceed to dispose of the water and subsequently relocate the bones to an alternative saucepan, preferably one with a greater capacity.
- Prior to incorporating it into the cooking vessel, divide the peeled onion in half and proceed to finely dice it. The subsequent procedure involves filling the container with water and integrating all of the substances that were considered optional but were ultimately chosen for inclusion. After the liquid has reached its boiling point, proceed to cover the pot with its lid and thereafter reduce the heat to a simmer.

- Once the mixture has been sieved into a new bowl, it should be allowed to cool to the ambient temperature prior to being covered and placed in the refrigerator. The resulting mixture will have a stratified composition, with a solidified substance forming an upper layer within a 24-hour period. This substance contains a high concentration of lipids, and it is advisable to remove as much of it as possible. The final product should possess a texture that is analogous to that of gelatin. Store the item in a freezer until it is ready for use.

90. Chicken Broth

Chicken broth is low in fat and calories and high in proteins, minerals, and vitamins. So it's a pretty good option for the clear liquid stage. This chicken broth (stock) recipe makes around six servings.

Ingredients:

- A large onion
- Water
- Two pounds of bony chicken meat
- Spring onions
- Ginger
- Carrot
- Garlic
- Thyme
- Rosemary
- Peppercorn

Directions:

- Put all of the Ingredients into a big saucepan and bring the pot to a low simmer. As soon as it reaches a boil, turn the heat down until the mixture is almost completely submerged in a barely perceptible pool of liquid. The Ingredients should be left to cook there without the cover on for between three and a half and four hours.

- Before proceeding to the next stage of the procedure, you will need to ensure that the mixture has cooled to room temperature. Once you have strained the stock into a larger bowl, separate the chicken meat from the bones and leave it aside. After you have done this, strain the stock again. This guarantees that not a single part of the chicken is thrown away. Place the bowl in the refrigerator, cover it, and let it sit cold for at least eight hours, or overnight. A lipid layer will develop on the surface of the broth. It is advisable to remove a significant portion of the layer of fat that accumulates on the surface of the soup.

91. Beef Broth

Beef broth is high in protein and fat and is nourishing and comforting for the body. It reduces inflammation and is great for our digestive health. It can be another option for the clear liquid stage. This yummy beef broth (stock) recipe makes around 10 servings.

Ingredients:

- A large onion
- Water
- Four pounds of bony beef meat
- Spring onions
- Ginger
- Carrot
- Garlic
- Thyme
- Rosemary
- Peppercorn
- Oregano
- Parsley
- Marjoram
- Celery

Direction:

- In the first step of the procedure, the oven needs to be preheated to a temperature of 450 degrees Fahrenheit. The last thirty minutes of the meat's cooking time in the roasting pan should be spent with the lid off. After the first half hour in the oven, add the veggies that have been chopped and continue baking for another half hour. Remove any excess fat that has formed on the surface of the contents of the roasting pan before placing the contents of the roasting pan into a Dutch oven.

- Put all of the Ingredients into a big saucepan and bring the pot to a low simmer. As soon as it reaches a boil, turn the heat down until the mixture is almost completely submerged in a barely perceptible pool of liquid. The Ingredients should be left to cook there without the cover on for between three and a half and four hours.

- Before we go on to the subsequent step, you will need to ensure that the mixture has cooled to room temperature. Once you have strained the stock into a larger bowl, separate the beef meat from the bones and leave it aside. After you have done this, strain the stock again. This guarantees that not a single part of the chicken is thrown away. Place the bowl in the refrigerator, cover it, and let it sit cold for at least eight hours, or overnight. A lipid layer will develop on the surface of the broth. It is advisable to remove a significant portion of the layer of fat that accumulates on the surface of the soup.

92. Ginger-Mushroom Broth

This high-protein, high-fibre broth is comforting and good for digestion. This recipe is for four servings.

Ingredients:

- A large onion
- Mushroom
- Water
- Spring onions
- Ginger
- Peppercorn
- Soy sauce
- Chicken broth

Directions:

- Put the ginger and mushrooms in the pot, then turn the heat up to medium-high and leave them like this for two minutes to allow them to cook. The next thing you need to do is bring it to a boil while simultaneously adding some soy sauce and chicken broth. Bring the mixture to a simmer over low heat and let it cook for a few minutes before adding the onion and basil.
- Remove any particles from the soup by straining it through a fine-mesh strainer, and then it's ready to be served!

93. Chicken Wonton Broth:

This high-protein, high-fibre broth is comforting and good for digestion. This recipe is for four servings.

The Ingredients are:

- A large onion
- Mushroom
- Water
- Spring onions
- Ginger
- Peppercorn

- Soy sauce
- Chicken broth
- Baby bok choy
- Sesame oil

Direction:

- Put some chicken broth into the pot, then bring it to a boil.
- Using a knife, crush the ginger, and then cut it into pieces.
- Put it in the saucepan and cover it with the lid when you've done so. Allow it to cook for a total of five minutes.
- After that, put the bok choy in the pan and let it cook for five minutes.
- After two to three minutes of simmering, add the mushrooms and wontons and cook until the mushrooms are soft and the wontons are wilted.
- Add the soy sauce and toasted sesame oil, and mix well.
- Pass the broth through a strainer to remove any solids.
- Serve, and have fun with it!

94. Chicken Consommé:

This dish is full of high protein and low carbs. It is really good for digestive health. It can be another option for the clear liquid stage. This yummy soup recipe makes around six servings.

Ingredients:

- celery
- Eight cups of chicken broth
- egg whites
- carrot
- chicken keema
- Salt

Direction:

- Place the chicken, celery, egg whites, and carrot in a pan that is approximately the size of a medium saucepan. They need to be mixed together, and then 2 cups of the chicken stock should be added while they are being stirred. After giving everything a good toss, pour in the remaining portion of the chicken stock and turn the heat up to high. While it is cooking, stir this mixture on a regular basis. After the components have begun to boil and a clear layer of sediment has formed atop the mixture, reduce the heat so that it maintains a moderate simmer for the next half an hour while the dish is being prepared.

- After forty-five minutes, take the saucepan off the burner and turn off the heat under the stove. To separate the clear liquid from the rest of the mixture, strain it through cheesecloth using a ladle. Repeat this step if any chunks of food remain in the liquid after the first straining. Put the consommé in the refrigerator and allow it to chill until a coating of fat forms on the surface. Take off this layer of fat and put the meat in the freezer until you're ready to use it.

95. Tomato Consommé:

This low-carb, high-fibre soup recipe is great for the digestive system. So this is a good option for the clear liquid stage.

Ingredients:
- basil leaves
- lemon
- garlic cloves
- tomatoes
- beetroot, sliced
- green onions
- black pepper
- kosher salt additionally
- cheesecloth

Direction:
- To achieve the required texture, combine lemon juice, green onions, tomatoes, garlic, basil, pepper, and kosher salt in the bowl of a food processor and process using intermittent pulses. Combine the Ingredients until they have a texture akin to that of ice cream. It is advisable to refrain from consuming this beverage at present since it does not possess desirable qualities for a smoothie. I can confidently assert this based on my personal experience and expertise in the matter. In a voluminous receptacle, arrange the limited number of cheesecloth pieces in a stack, ensuring that they are organized in ascending order based on their size.

- Subsequently, the tomato mixture should be poured over the aforementioned components. Grasp the four corners of the cheesecloth and elevate them, enveloping the mixture within the confines of a cheesecloth bag. Subsequently, remove the cheesecloth from the base of the bowl. Once the four corners of the cheesecloth have been securely fastened, proceed to incorporate the beetroot into the bowl, as this will impart the desired hue to the combination. Subsequently, suspend the compact cheesecloth pouch over the bowl in a manner that ensures its complete coverage, and place the ensemble within the refrigerator. In a literal interpretation, the sole requirement is to elevate the bag over the bowl for many hours, facilitating the complete filtration of the mixture through it. Once the combination has been sufficiently strained, it is permissible to discard both the cheesecloth bag and the beetroot residue located at the bottom of the container. When dispensing liquid or semi-liquid substances, it is recommended to employ a ladle.

96. Vegetable Consommé

This low-carb and high-fibre soup recipe is great for the digestive system. So this can be a good option for the clear liquid stage.

Ingredients:

- basil leaves
- lemon
- Turnips
- Potatoes
- garlic cloves
- tomatoes
- beetroot, sliced
- green onions
- black pepper
- kosher salt additionally
- cheesecloth

Direction:

- To achieve the required texture, combine all the Ingredients, along with kosher salt, in the bowl of a food processor and process using intermittent pulses. Combine the Ingredients until they have a texture akin to that of ice cream. It is advisable to refrain from consuming this beverage at present since it does not possess desirable qualities for a smoothie. I can confidently assert this based on my personal experience and expertise in the matter.

- In a voluminous receptacle, arrange the limited number of cheesecloth pieces in a stack, ensuring that they are organised in ascending order based on their size.

- Subsequently, the tomato mixture should be poured over the aforementioned components. Grasp the four corners of the cheesecloth and elevate them, enveloping the mixture within the confines of a cheesecloth bag. Subsequently, remove the cheesecloth from the base of the bowl. Once the four corners of the cheesecloth have been securely fastened, proceed to incorporate the beetroot into the bowl, as this will impart the desired hue to the combination. Subsequently, suspend the compact cheesecloth pouch over the bowl in a manner that ensures its complete coverage, and place the ensemble within the refrigerator. In a literal interpretation, the sole requirement is to elevate the bag over the bowl for many hours, facilitating the complete filtration of the mixture through it. Once the combination has been sufficiently strained, it is permissible to discard both the cheesecloth bag and the beetroot residue located at the bottom of the container. When dispensing liquid or semi-liquid substances, it is recommended to employ a ladle.

97. Poached Black Sesame Salmon and Bok Choy Broth:

Ingredients:
- Pickles liquid
- Black pepper
- Red cabbage, chopped
- Onion (1 pc.)
- Lemon (1 pc.)
- Zucchini (2.)
- White wine (1 cup)
- Liquid (2 cups)
- kosher-salt
- Cayenne pepper

Direction:
- Preheat the broiler to 400°F. Strip and cut the yams into tiny pieces.
- Put the yams on a baking sheet and toss them with pepper.
- Olive oil and salt. Cook the potatoes in the broiler for 45–50 minutes at 400°F, or until the yams are very caramelised. Put away.
- In an enormous soup pot, cook the leeks or onions over medium-high heat for 8 minutes or until they are delicate Stir in the garlic and ginger, then continue cooking for a second. Add the white wine and heat it to the point of boiling until the wine vanishes.
- Whenever all the wine has dissipated, add the vegetable stock, thyme, and yams, and at that point, bring the entire soup blend into a bubble. Turn down the heat and let it stew for 20 minutes, or until the vegetables are delicate, if necessary.
- Utilise a blender to puree the soup in clusters. Warm each group of soups prior to serving.

98. Kanji

It is an Indian probiotic drink that is great for the digestive system and reduces inflammation.

Ingredients:
- Brown Mustard Seeds
- carrots
- beet
- salt
- Sugar

Method:
- To grind the mustard seeds, you can either use a mortar and pestle or a coffee grinder; coarse grinding is acceptable.
- Carrots and beets should be cut into long, chunky pieces.
- Combine all of the Ingredients in a jar made of glass. Cover it with a lid or a piece of cheesecloth, and place it on top.
- Allow the jar to sit in a bright place for at least a week while stirring the contents of it with a wooden spoon on a daily basis.
- When the kanji starts to have a sour flavour, the drink has finished fermenting.
- Put the pickles in a separate container for later use, and strain the juice.
- Put the beverage in the refrigerator to get it nice and cold.

99. Spicy Lemonade

This drink is full of vitamins and refreshing.

Ingredients:
- Water
- Sugar
- Salt
- Lime
- Black salt
- Mint leaves
- Ice cube

Method:

- Thoroughly combine all of the Ingredients in the mixture. Taste the dish to determine the appropriate amounts of sweetness, sourness, salt, and Indian black salt to add. (At this point, the combination can be stored in the refrigerator for up to two days to be refrigerated.)

- After placing ice cubes in the cups, proceed with the service. For garnish, try some lime slices or mint leaves.. Please refer to the notes for any variations.

100. Ginger juice

This drink is really refreshing. It's good for digestive health.

Ingredients:

- Water
- Ginger root
- Salt
- Lime
- Chaat Masala
- Black salt
- Mint leaves
- Ice cube

Method:

- Thoroughly combine all of the Ingredients in the mixture. Taste the dish to determine the appropriate amounts of sourness, salt, and Indian black salt to add. (At this point, the combination can be stored in the refrigerator for up to two days to be refrigerated.)

- After placing ice cubes in the cups, proceed with the service. For garnish, try some lime slices or mint leaves.. Please refer to the notes for any variations.

101. Fruit Punch

A fruit punch has both sour and sweet flavours, and it is typically a transparent drink. This fruit punch recipe will make enough for around 20 servings, so plan accordingly.

Ingredients:

- water
- strawberries,
- orange juice
- Sprite or other lemon-lime soda
- Pineapple juice

- 2 6-ounce cans of thawed lemonade concentrate
- sugar

Direction:

- Combine the orange juice and lemonade concentrates, as well as the pineapple juice, in a large container and thoroughly mix the contents. Bring the remaining sugar and water to a boil and continue to cook for about 5 minutes, or until the sugar is completely dissolved. After that, place the sliced strawberries in a ring mould, add enough fruit juice to completely fill the mould, and freeze the mould.

- Place any remaining juice in the bottle in the refrigerator. When you're ready to serve it to your guests, combine all of the **Ingredients:** in a suitable container and top with Sprite. The last step is to place the frozen strawberry ring in the basin.

102. Vegetable Juice

Vegetable juice has a refreshing flavour.

Ingredients:

- Carrots
- Water
- Bellpepper
- Celery
- Lime juice
- Onion
- Salt
- Serrano pepper

Direction:

- Incorporate a measured amount of water along with bell pepper, Serrano pepper, celery and carrots, lime juice, onion, and salt into the Dutch oven. The stems and seeds should be removed from the serrano peppers. After that, put everything in the Dutch oven. Let the water boil.

- Subsequently, decrease the boiling point to a gentle simmer and continue cooking for an additional duration of thirty minutes, or until the veggies have reached a state of tenderness.

- Allow it to cool down.

- Pour the mixture into the serving glasses after straining it through the strainer.

- Serve, and have fun with it!

103. Carrot and orange juice:

It's a very refreshing drink. So, it can be added to the list of recipes for the clear liquid stage.

Ingredients:

- Carrots
- Oranges

Direction:

- To begin, the carrots need to be peeled, trimmed, and brushed before being added to the blender.
- Add the oranges that have been peeled and mix until smooth.
- Remove any solid bits from the juice by straining it through a fine mesh sieve.
- Serve, and have fun with it!

104. Cranberry Juice

It can be an excellent option for a clear liquid stage.

Ingredients::

- Cranberries
- water
- Lemon juice
- Honey

Direction:

- In a blender, combine the water and cranberries for two minutes at high speed. Blend until smooth.
- Remove any particles from the juice by straining it through a fine-mesh strainer or cheesecloth.
- Mix honey and lemon juice into the juice and set it aside.
- When you are finished, transfer the mixture to the glasses.

105. White Grape Juice

Ingredients::
- White grapes
- Water
- Ginger root
- Salt
- Lime
- Ice cubes

Direction:
- Place the ginger, sugar, grapes, lemon juice, and salt in the container of a blender.
- Start the blender. Combine until there are no lumps.
- Pour the juice through a sieve, and throw away the pulp and other solids.
- Place several ice cubes in the serving glass, and then pour some juice into the glass. Serve, and have fun with it!

106. Pineapple juice

This drink is refreshing and delicious. It's quite a convenient option for the clear liquid stage.

Ingredients:
- Water
- Ginger root
- Salt
- Black pepper
- Pineapple

Direction:
- To begin, remove both of the pineapple's ends and set them aside.
- Using a knife that is somewhat sharp, cut the pineapple skin into pieces.
- Place the pineapple chunks in the blender along with the rest of the Ingredients.
- Blend until there are no lumps.
- Remove any solid particles from the juice by straining it through a fine-mesh sieve.
- Serve, and have fun with it!

107. Apple Juice

Apple juice helps clean the colon by breaking down toxins and improving liver and bowel movement. So it's a good option for the clear liquid stage.

Ingredients:
- Apple
- Sugar

Direction:
- The apples need to be washed and peeled before they can be used. It needs to be divided into smaller pieces.
- Remove the seeds from the fruit.
- Place apple slices and sugar in the juicer, and run it through the machine until the liquid becomes clear.
- Serve, and don't forget to have fun doing it!

108. Honey Lemon Tea

This delicious hot drink is a great breakfast option for patients in the clear liquid stage.

Ingredients:
- Water
- Back tea
- Lemon juice
- Honey

Direction:
- Put some water in the pot and start heating it up.
- Bring it to a simmer, and then stir in the tea leaves. Allow the mixture to sit for one minute. Pour the tea into the serving cups after straining it through the filter.
- Combine the honey and lemon juice in a mixing bowl and stir until combined.
- Serve, and have fun with it!

109. Ginger Tea

It's a comfy hot drink that feels like a warm hug.

Ingredients:

- Water
- Black tea
- Ginger

Direction:

- To get started, fill the saucepan with water and ginger that has been shredded. After that, raise the temperature to the level that you want it to be at.
- After the water has been heated to a low simmer, the tea leaves should be put into the vessel where they will steep. After letting the Ingredients rest for a minute, give the mixture one more toss in order to combine everything. After the tea has been poured through the filter, it should be poured into the cups that are going to be used for serving.
- If you are going to be of service to others, don't forget to take care of yourself so that you can enjoy the experience!

110. Iced Sweet Tea

This sweet and refreshing drink is great for digestive health.

Ingredients:

- Tea bags
- Sugar
- Water
- Ice
- Lemon
- Mint leaves

Direction:

- Bring the equivalent of four cups of water to a boil in a saucepan. After that, remove the pot from the heat and add the tea bags.
- To ensure that the bags have the opportunity to completely absorb the water, you will need to submerge and remove them from the water several times. Give the tea bags about five minutes to steep in the water before removing them. After five minutes, take the bags out of the freezer and throw them away. After adding the sugar to the liquid, make sure to give it a good stir to ensure that it is completely dissolved.
- Obtain your pitcher or any suitable container in which you intend to store the tea, and pour the tea into it. Because the tea you just produced is so strong, you need to dilute it with

another 12 cups of water before serving it. Pour the water into the pitcher. The trick to adequately chilling the tea and serving it over ice is to hold off on adding this water until later on in the process.

- It is recommended that you place this in the refrigerator the previous night so that it can be served at a very chilly temperature. If you truly don't want to have to wait that long, then you only need to wait for four hours. When you are ready to serve the beverage, put a ton of ice in it, and if you think it would taste well with some, serve it with a few mint leaves or a slice of lemon.

111. Cranberry iced green tea

It is made with cranberry juice and green tea, and it's a very refreshing drink.

Ingredients:
- Green tea bags
- Cranberry juice
- Hot water
- Watermelon wedges
- Orange slices
- mint

Direction:
- Put an entire cup of cranberry juice into the ice cube tray, and then place the tray in the freezer to chill.
- Once the water has boiled, insert the tea bags into it and allow it to cool down before removing them.
- Toss the used tea bags into the garbage. Add the cranberry juice to the bowl, and whisk the Ingredients together until they are fully incorporated.
- Fill each of the four cups with cranberry-flavoured ice cubes that you have already prepared. After that, place a slice of orange and a watermelon wedge on top of the watermelon wedge.
- Add some cranberry tea to each of the serving cups by pouring it in.
- Garnish with some freshly chopped mint!

112. Black tea

Ingredients:
- Tea
- Sugar
- Water

Direction:
- After you have added some water to the pan, you should put it on the stove over high heat so that the liquid can boil.
- After that, pour in the tea, and then immediately remove the pot from the flame to put an end to the process of heating it.
- When you have finished covering the pot with the lid, place it on a surface that can bear heat and wait for approximately two to three minutes after doing so.
- After the sugar has been dissolved into the beverage, the tea must first be poured into the pitcher before being transferred to individual glasses for consumption.
- While you're serving others, don't forget to take some time out to enjoy yourself.

113. Spicy Milk Tea

Ingredients:
- Oat milk
- Ginger
- Cinnamon sticks
- Cloves
- Tea

Direction:
- To get things rolling, put some water in a pot and bring it to a simmer over medium heat. This will get things off to a good start. The tea leaves, water, sugar, ginger, and cinnamon sticks should all be placed inside the container. You could also put in some ground ginger and cloves.
- Between eight and nine minutes is the normal amount of time needed for water to reach a complete rolling boil after being brought to a boil.
- When you're adding the oat milk, do so in a stream that is both extremely slow and very careful. After around eight to ten minutes, the liquid should be quite close to the point where it will boil.
- It is recommended that as soon as the mixture has been poured into the cup and sifted, it be served.

114. Turmeric Milk Tea

Ingredients:
- Water
- Ginger tea bags (3)
- Oat milk (3 cups)
- Ground cinnamon
- Ground turmeric
- Ground ginger
- Honey

Direction:
- In a medium bowl, pour the water over your tea bags.
- Then, steep them for around 5 minutes.
- Later, remove your tea bags & combine oat milk, ginger, cinnamon, turmeric, & honey.
- Transfer mixture to your blender & blend for around 20 seconds.
- Divide your golden milk tea among 5 glasses.
- Serve it.
- Enjoy!

A 30 DAYS MEAL PLAN

1ST 10 DAYS	2ND 10 DAYS	3RD 10 DAYS
DAY-1	**DAY-11**	**DAY-21**
Breakfast: Delicious Oatmeal with Turmeric Powder **Lunch:** LOW-FIBER Omelet **Dinner:** Banana Almond Milk Smoothie	**Breakfast:** Turmeric Milk Tea **Lunch:** Banana and Almond Butter Oatmeal **Dinner:** Baked Spaghetti Squash with Parmesan Cheese	**Breakfast:** Green Tea and Ginger Shake **Lunch:** Salad with Kale, Onions, and Apple Cider Vinegar **Dinner:** Homemade Chocolate Ice Cream
DAY-2	**DAY-12**	**DAY-22**
Breakfast: Turmeric Milk Tea **Lunch:** Banana and Almond Butter Oatmeal **Dinner:** Baked Spaghetti Squash with Parmesan Cheese	**Breakfast:** Blueberry smoothie **Lunch:** Ginger Carrot Soup with Turmeric Powder **Dinner:** Bone Broth	**Breakfast:** Blueberry-Millet Breakfast Bake **Lunch:** Flax-Almond Porridge **Dinner:** Chicken Wonton Broth
DAY-3	**DAY-13**	**DAY-23**
Breakfast: Low-fiber banana smoothie **Lunch:** Anti-Inflammatory Stir-fry **Dinner:** Poached Black Sesame Salmon and Bok Choy Broth	**Breakfast:** Blueberry-Millet Breakfast Bake **Lunch:** Flax-Almond Porridge **Dinner:** Chicken Wonton Broth	**Breakfast:** COCONUT pudding **Lunch:** Baked Salmon with Rosemary and Lemon **Dinner:** Spicy Milk Tea
DAY-4	**DAY-14**	**DAY-24**
Breakfast: Smoked Turkey-Wrapped Zucchini Sticks **Lunch:** Applesauce Burger with Spinach Salad **Dinner:** Apple Juice	**Breakfast:** Delicious Oatmeal with Turmeric Powder **Lunch:** LOW-FIBER Omelet **Dinner:** Banana Almond Milk Smoothie	**Breakfast:** Cucumber and Smoked-Salmon Lettuce Wraps **Lunch:** BUTTERNUT Coconut Red Lentil Soup **Dinner:** Honey Lemon Tea

DAY-5	DAY-15	DAY-25
Breakfast: Blueberry-Millet Breakfast Bake **Lunch:** Flax-Almond Porridge **Dinner:** Chicken Wonton Broth	**Breakfast:** Blackened Chicken Avocado Power Bowl **Lunch:** CHICKEN Adobo **Dinner:** Cranberry iced green tea	**Breakfast:** Blueberry smoothie **Lunch:** Ginger Carrot Soup with Turmeric Powder **Dinner:** Bone Broth
DAY-6	**DAY-16**	**DAY-26**
Breakfast: Green Tea and Ginger Shake **Lunch:** Salad with Kale, Onions, and Apple Cider Vinegar **Dinner:** Homemade Chocolate Ice Cream	**Breakfast:** Smoked Turkey-Wrapped Zucchini Sticks **Lunch:** Applesauce Burger with Spinach Salad **Dinner:** Apple Juice	**Breakfast:** Low-fiber banana smoothie **Lunch:** Anti-Inflammatory Stir-fry **Dinner:** Poached Black Sesame Salmon and Bok Choy Broth
DAY-7	**DAY-17**	**DAY-27**
Breakfast: Blueberry smoothie **Lunch:** Ginger Carrot Soup with Turmeric Powder **Dinner:** Bone Broth	**Breakfast:** Cucumber and Smoked-Salmon Lettuce Wraps **Lunch:** BUTTERNUT Coconut Red Lentil Soup **Dinner:** Honey Lemon Tea	**Breakfast:** COCONUT pudding **Lunch:** Baked Salmon with Rosemary and Lemon **Dinner:** Spicy Milk Tea
DAY-8	**DAY-18**	**DAY-28**
Breakfast: COCONUT pudding **Lunch:** Baked Salmon with Rosemary and Lemon **Dinner:** Spicy Milk Tea	**Breakfast:** Low-fiber banana smoothie **Lunch:** Anti-Inflammatory Stir-fry **Dinner:** Poached Black Sesame Salmon and Bok Choy Broth	**Breakfast:** Turmeric Milk Tea **Lunch:** Banana and Almond Butter Oatmeal **Dinner:** Baked Spaghetti Squash with Parmesan Cheese

DAY-9	**DAY-19**	**DAY-29**
Breakfast: Cucumber and Smoked-Salmon Lettuce Wraps **Lunch:** BUTTERNUT Coconut Red Lentil Soup **Dinner:** Honey Lemon Tea	**Breakfast:** Blackened Chicken Avocado Power Bowl **Lunch:** CHICKEN Adobo **Dinner:** Cranberry iced green tea	**Breakfast:** Smoked Turkey-Wrapped Zucchini Sticks **Lunch:** Applesauce Burger with Spinach Salad **Dinner:** Apple Juice
DAY-10	**DAY-20**	**DAY-30**
Breakfast: Green Tea and Ginger Shake **Lunch:** Salad with Kale, Onions, and Apple Cider Vinegar **Dinner:** Homemade Chocolate Ice Cream	**Breakfast:** Blackened Chicken Avocado Power Bowl **Lunch:** CHICKEN Adobo **Dinner:** Cranberry iced green tea	**Breakfast:** Delicious Oatmeal with Turmeric Powder **Lunch:** LOW-FIBER Omelet **Dinner:** Banana Almond Milk Smoothie

Conclusion

Foods that have a significant amount of dietary fibre integrated into their overall chemical composition are called high-fibre foods. The high quantities of dietary fibre and other beneficial nutrients that can be found in products like bread produced with whole wheat and other meals manufactured with whole grains have helped make these products immensely popular. Other foods manufactured with whole grains also include high levels of these nutrients. In addition to this, it is extremely recommended that bran be incorporated into a person's diet on a regular basis so that it can serve as a component of that diet. This category contains fermented greens like sauerkraut as well as fermented legumes that have not been entirely cooked or are just partially cooked. Examples of foods in this category include sauerkraut and kimchi. It is suggested to consume fresh fruits and vegetables without peeling them since this enables the consumption of them in their natural condition and ensures the consumption of dietary fibre, which is absent in juices.

Following the meal, a selection of snacks and beverages are made available for consumption. People who have diverticulitis may have a lower projected lifespan, a higher chance of developing cardiovascular diseases, and the possible need for interventions for more serious difficulties, such as surgical operations. This is because diverticulitis can cause inflammation of the diverticulum, which can cause inflammation of the colon. In addition, those who have diverticulitis may have a higher risk of developing issues that are connected to their digestive system.

Patients and medical professionals both have an interest in locating pharmaceutical therapies that have a chance of successfully lowering the risk of developing cardiovascular syndrome or diverticulitis. This is a goal that both groups have in common. Modifications to a person's way of life, such as modifications to their nutrition, are of utmost importance as potential strategies for enhancing their health and well-being. When it comes to the condition of diverticulitis, this holds true not just for patients, but also for the attending physicians who take care of them. Individuals now have the capability, as a further consequence of these enhancements, to engage in "self-management of their diverticulitis disease treatment." It is recommended that people who have been diagnosed with diverticulitis make changes to their diets, since this is recommended by empirical data acquired from both individuals and research that was not conducted using a randomized design. Individuals who have been diagnosed with diverticulitis should consider making changes to their diets. According to the findings of these studies, making some relatively little alterations to a person's typical diet has the potential to lessen the likelihood of that person suffering a heart attack as well as the general mortality rate in a population as a whole.

Made in the USA
Coppell, TX
15 January 2025